PENGUIN BOOKS

# FOOD FOR THOUGHT

David Benton was born in 1947 in Newcastle upon Tyne and he
received his doctorate from the University of Birmingham in 1974 for
research examining the relationship between brain chemistry and
behaviour. He is currently Reader in Psychology at the University of
Wales, Swansea. For over ten years he has examined the impact of
diet on behaviour, research that has considered our intake of vitamins,
minerals and fat and the influence of diet-induced changes in blood
glucose. In many dozens of research papers he has reported that diet
influences mood, memory, attention and intelligence, findings that
have attracted widespread media attention.

# FOOD FOR THOUGHT

*How what you eat affects your*
*mood, memory and thinking*

## David Benton

PENGUIN BOOKS

PENGUIN BOOKS

Published by the Penguin Group
Penguin Books Ltd, 27 Wrights Lane, London w8 5TZ, England
Penguin Books USA Inc., 375 Hudson Street, New York, New York 10014, USA
Penguin Books Australia Ltd, Ringwood, Victoria, Australia
Penguin Books Canada Ltd, 10 Alcorn Avenue, Toronto, Ontario, Canada M4V 3B2
Penguin Books (NZ) Ltd, 182–190 Wairau Road, Auckland 10, New Zealand

Penguin Books Ltd, Registered Offices: Harmondsworth, Middlesex, England

First published 1996
1 3 5 7 9 10 8 6 4 2

The acknowledgements on p. vi constitute an
extension of this copyright page

Figures drawn by Nigel Andrews

Set in 10.25/12.5 Monotype Ehrhardt
Typeset by Datix International Limited, Bungay, Suffolk
Printed in England by Clays Ltd, St Ives plc

# Contents

# Acknowledgements

The author and publisher are grateful to the following sources for their kind permission to use copyright material. Every effort has been made to obtain permission for the use of copyright material, and acknowledgements have also been given throughout the book. If notified of any errors or omissions, the publisher will be happy to make corrections in the next edition.

Fig. 3.2, Z. A. Stein *et al.*, *Famine and Human Development: the Dutch Hunger Winter of 1944/45*, 1975, by permission of Oxford University Press; Fig. 3.5, Data from A. Lucas, R. Morley, T. J. Cole, G. Lister and Leeson-Payne, 'Breast milk and subsequent intelligence quotient in children born preterm', *Lancet*, 339, 1992, 261–4; Fig. 4.4, D. Benton and G. Roberts, 'Effect of vitamin and mineral supplementation on intelligence of a sample of schoolchildren', *Lancet*, i, 1988, 140–43, © by The Lancet Ltd, 1988; Table 5.2, 'Food Intolerance and Food Aversion', *Journal of the Royal College of Physicians*, 18, 1984, 1–41; Table 6.1, reproduced with permission from G. Cannon, *The Politics of Food*, Century, 1987; Table 6.3, J. Egger *et al.*, 'Controlled trial of olioantigenic treatment in the hyperkinetic syndrome', *Lancet*, 14, 1985, 540–45, Table V, © by The Lancet Ltd, 1985; Fig. 7.5, J. Keul *et al.*, 'Einfluss von Dextrose auf Fahrleistung, Konzentrationsfahigkeit, Kreislauf und Stoffwechsel im Kraftfahrzeug-Simulator (Doppelblindstudie im cross-over-design), *Akt. Erhähr.* 7 (1982) 7–14 Georg Thieme Verlag; Fig. 10.3, reprinted from *Experimental Gerontology*, 24, S. N. Austrad, 'Life extension by dietary restriction in the bowl and doily spider, *Frontinella pyramitela*', 83–92, Copyright 1989, with kind permission from Elsevier Science Ltd, The Boulevard, Langford Lane, Kidlington OX5 1GB UK; Fig. 11.2, reprinted by permission of the publisher from Fig. 2, D. J. Bowen and N. E. Grunberg, 'Variation in food preference and consumption across the menstrual cycle', *Physiology and Behavior*, 47, 287–91, Copyright 1990 by Elsevier Science Inc.; Fig. 11.3, reprinted by permission of the publisher from Fig. 2, S. P. Dalvit-McPhillips, 'The effect of the human menstrual cycle on nutrient intake', *Physiology and Behavior*, 31, 209–12, Copyright 1983 by Elsevier Science Inc.; Fig. 12.2, S. Folkard and T. H. Monk (eds.), *Hours of Work: Temporal Factors in Work Scheduling*, fig. 19.2, © Folkard and Monk, 1985, reprinted by permission of John Wiley & Sons Ltd.

# *Preface*

It is difficult for somebody who is academically trained to write for a general audience. There is a widespread view in academic circles that if you try to communicate with the general population, the inevitable simplification amounts to being inaccurate and hence misleading. In fact, in academic circles it is too easy to be totally destructive by listing the multitude of problems of interpretation that arise when any topic is considered. Only too often the strict scientific conclusion is that nothing can be said with certainty. If you can say something, then it applies only to a highly selected group of people, with a very specific diet, of a certain age; you cannot generalize to other people in other situations. Taking an extreme scientific viewpoint risks finding that it is unreasonable to come to any conclusion; no general advice can be offered.

Such an approach, although valid in its own terms, when taken in a wider perspective can be unhelpful. We may rarely even approach 100 per cent scientific certainty, but many scientists are paid out of public funds to help inform the public about matters of general concern. The aim is to examine such concerns and offer advice.

If certainty cannot be offered, then an informed opinion is of value. It is in this spirit that the book is written. The possibility that diet may influence the way we feel, think and behave has on numerous occasions been a matter for public concern, but we can say little about it with total confidence. The nature of the available evidence and the associated problems will be outlined. Whereas when wearing a scientific hat I can rarely come off the fence and offer guidance, here, in contrast, I have tried to offer considered advice for those who might be concerned about what they eat.

There is no doubt that the approach will be criticized from at least two perspectives. Scientists may feel that I have, on occasion, gone beyond the data in drawing conclusions. They may well be correct, but I have attempted to indicate when I have done this and why. A book that lists scientific ignorance without even tentative conclusions is of little value to people who wish to provide themselves and their family with a good diet. I hope the book is viewed in this light by my academic colleagues. At the other end of the spectrum I have little doubt that many people who believe that diet is a widespread cause of problems will view my comments as too negative and too conservative. The conclusion that the weight of evidence indicates that many dietary 'cures' do not work will prove unwelcome. I trust that in between these two groups there is an audience without too many preconceptions, who will judge the book in the spirit intended.

# CHAPTER I

# Are You What You Eat?

In recent years there has been an explosion of interest in the possibility that what you eat may influence the way you think and feel. Often claims are of a sensational nature, implying that aspects of diet are both the cause and the means of solving complex and worrying problems:

... millions may be made ill, physically and mentally, by common foods such as milk, eggs, coffee and white flour;[1]

For one person in every ten, sugar is a deadly food, paving the way towards a hundred distressing physical symptoms, plus all the tortures of neurotic and even psychotic symptoms;[2]

... Factors believed to contribute to the etiology of hyperactivity include ingestion of artificial food additives such as colors and flavors;[3]

Feed your kids a better IQ;[4]

Senility is a form of malnutrition – and can be avoided, or even reversed, by sound nutritional planning.[5]

While there may be some basis for such statements, usually only more limited assertions can be justified. Frequently, behind the questionable headlines there are questionable scientific studies, and claims are based on limited, over-generalized findings or even anecdotal comments. None the less it should not be assumed that diet is never of dramatic importance or that we are not all influenced in subtle ways. Diet may influence behaviour, but it is simply one of many factors that do, and only on rare occasions is it likely to predominate.

## *Will anything cure the sick?*

Throughout history the physician has held a respected place in society, although for the majority of that time there were on offer few, if any, useful treatments. Charles II, being the king of England, had the services of the best doctors, and this was how he was treated:

A pint of blood was extracted from his right shoulder, followed by an emetic, two physics, and an enema comprising fifteen substances; the royal head was then shaved and a blister raised; then a sneezing powder, more emetics and bleeding, soothing potions, a plaster of pitch and pigeon dung on his feet, potions containing ten different substances, chiefly herbs, finally forty drops of extract of human skull, and the application of bezoar stone; after which his majesty died.[6]

In ancient Egypt medicines included lizards' blood, crocodile dung, putrid meat and fly droppings. In other places and at other times the flesh of vipers, spermatic fluid of frogs, holy oil, powdered Egyptian mummy, eunuch fat and usnea (moss scraped from the skull of a hanged criminal) have been the 'medicines' of choice.[7]

Although Charles II would have had grounds for complaining to the General Medical Council, it is reasonable to assume that physicians must have helped at least some patients, as they maintained their position in society over many centuries. How did they manage to do this using treatments that were at the best useless and at worst dangerous? The answer is that any treatment, especially a new, expensive, unusual or unpleasant one, will generate a placebo response.

The term placebo means that the treatment has no intrinsic pharmacological activity, and that any response is psychological in nature, a reflection of expectation, faith and suggestion. There is nothing wrong with a placebo response – in fact, it's a major weapon in the doctor's armoury – but it is important to distinguish active treatments so patients can be offered the additional benefit.

If we change our diet or take a vitamin supplement there will be an inevitable psychological benefit; as the history of medicine shows, responses occur to the most unlikely substances. In 1959 the *Journal of the American Medical Association* noted that at that time approximately 10 per cent of medical expenses in the United States were spent on vitamins, 'which are often prescribed both knowingly and unknowingly for their placebo effect'.[8] Whereas the general public seems readily prepared to believe that diet can both cause and cure a multitude of problems, such suggestions generate considerable scepticism, if not hostility, in much of the medical profession. Many doctors and professional nutritionists are certain that the diet in industrialized societies is adequate. Any supposed benefits of an altered diet are explained away, with little if any consideration, as the psychological response of the unsophisticated and gullible. Professor Vincent Marks, a biochemist at the University of Surrey, reflected the views of many of his colleagues when he said:

Healthy people do not need vitamin supplements. However poor an individual's diet might be, it is unlikely to cause a vitamin deficiency disease ... vitamin supplements, potentially dangerous if taken in overdoses, should carry health warnings like tobacco ... My belief is that anyone who needs vitamins needs to see a doctor. If they need supplements it will be because they have something wrong with them which affects the ability of the gut to absorb essential nutrients.[9]

There is truth in many of the details of this statement, but do they tell the whole story? Although many people are well nourished, some are not. And while it is extremely unlikely that the latter are so poorly nourished that they will have a vitamin deficiency disease, more minor deficiencies can, as we shall see, have psychological consequences.

## Old ideas

The belief in the importance of diet for good health and as a means of manipulating behaviour has a long history. The ancient Egyptians believed that salt would stimulate passion, that onions would induce sleep, and that cabbage and almonds would prevent drunkenness when drinking alcohol. The Greeks subscribed to the doctrine that the human temperament could be divided into the sanguine, the melancholic, the choleric and the phlegmatic, according to the dominance of the four basic humours in the body: red blood, black bile, yellow bile and phlegm. The consumption of various foods was said to change the combination of the basic humours, correct the balance between them, and thus alter an individual's personality.

John Harvey Kellogg, remembered today as the founder of a firm that produces breakfast cereals, was a leading light in the nineteenth-century health reform movement in the United States. He wrote and lectured widely, promoting the use of natural foods. He argued against the eating of meat, which he believed would arouse animal passion and cause symptoms that included depression, fatigue, aggression and mental illness: 'The secret of nine-tenths of all chronic ills from which civilized human beings suffer' ranging from 'national inefficiency' to 'Moral and social maladies' can be traced to the meat eater's sluggish bowels.[10]

Similar beliefs about the influence that diet has on behaviour are widely held today; they are not merely historical curiosities. While a great many people occasionally look at food labels to avoid additives, a few do so to such an extent that their attitude may be viewed as unreasonable or an example of food faddism. In fact it is possible to make a living by offering fringe medicinal procedures based on changing diet and prescribing vitamins and minerals.

Table 1.1 lists some distinguishing features of a food faddist or quack, who can be defined as somebody with an exaggerated belief in the importance of diet in health and disease. Typically, the nutritional benefits of various foods are overemphasized – raw foods, whole grains and organic foods are three common examples – while the effects of some constituents of natural and prepared foods, such as caffeine, sugar and food additives, cause apprehension. Although such views may be benign, in some instances they can have serious consequences. To be healthy, people need to eat a nutritious diet, one that provides sufficient quantities of protein, carbohydrate, fats, vitamins and minerals (see Chapter 2). People who eat a very unusual diet that is not based on adequate nutritional

*Table 1.1* **How to spot a food faddist and quack**

---

1 There are promises of rapid miraculous cures.

2 Personal experience and testimonials are used to justify claims.

3 A series of degrees, diplomas and other credentials from obscure schools without academic accreditation are displayed on the wall and quoted on letter headings.

4 Problems are diagnosed using tests that are not used by the medical profession and lack a suitable background of scientific evaluation.

5 You are told that knowledge of the benefits of the nutritional approach are being intentionally suppressed for the financial gain of the medical profession and pharmaceutical industry.

6 Sales are offered directly to the public often through advertisements in magazines rather than via a doctor or pharmacist.

7 They charge large fees for their nutritional products and consultations.

---

*Sources:* Adapted from W. T. Jarvis, 'Food faddism, cultism and quackery', *Annual Review of Nutrition*, 3, 1983, 35–52; V. Herbert and S. Barrett, 'Twenty-one ways to spot a quack', *Nutrition Forum Newsletter*, Sept. 1986, 65–8.

knowledge face the danger that it is unbalanced, that it does not supply sufficient quantities of all the nutrients they need. In 1985 Professor Marks coined the phrase 'muesli-belt malnutrition' to describe the nutritional problems of affluent people caused by the decision to eat an unusual, quirky and unbalanced diet.

Some, but not all, vitamins, if taken in excess, can produce adverse effects; too much vitamin A, for example, can cause nausea and vomiting. A large dose of some minerals can deplete the body of others and result in a deficiency; a large dose of zinc, for example, will deplete the body of copper, which can cause anaemia, irritability and the loss of the sense of taste. A range of nutritional deficiencies has been associated with extreme vegetarian diets, including rickets[11] and pernicious anaemia.[12] The case study of Frances shows that iron deficiency can be a problem for those eating a vegetarian diet. Vegetarian diets do not inevitably lead to nutritional problems – in fact vegetarians are less likely to suffer from a range of diseases – but they require background knowledge and appropriate planning. Care should be taken that any diet is well balanced; it is perhaps easier for novel diets to cause problems than solve them.

---

### Frances: problems of a thoughtless vegetarian

Frances was preparing to take the examinations that she needed to pass in order to go to university. She was finding revision very difficult; she was pale, had little energy, wanted to sleep much of the time and had problems concentrating. Her mother made her an appointment with the doctor. A blood test revealed that Frances had anaemia; her iron level was low and her body had no reserves of this mineral. For this reason she was given iron injections. Over several weeks her colour returned and she regained her energy.

The problem had been caused by Frances becoming a vegetarian without giving it much thought. Vegetarianism had become very popular in her circle of friends and Frances had vague worries about the impact of meat on health and ethical concerns about farming methods. Although her parents were happy for her to be a vegetarian, they made it clear that they were not going to cook two different meals every night. She was told that she would have to take responsibility for at least part of her meals, something she did not do. Instead, she simply ate the family meal without any meat. The result was that she became anaemic. This episode, in which the levels of haemoglobin in her blood had become so low that the doctor said that there was a risk of heart failure, forced Frances to take seriously her decision to be a vegetarian. She read books and learned of the need to eat a varied diet. She learned which foods contained iron and that although iron from plant sources is poorly absorbed by the human body, taking vitamin C can improve its uptake.

---

## Good scientific evidence

In examining suggestions that aspects of diet might influence our mood and the way we think, the powerful nature of the placebo response makes anecdotal comments or the response of a single individual a poor source of information. When one person claims that his or her problem has either been caused or cured by a change in diet, there is no way of knowing if anything other than a placebo response is involved. Scientists with a closed mind, who believe that an active response is unlikely, or even impossible, will, without giving the matter serious consideration, explain it away as a placebo response. Open-minded scientists will treat such claims as an interesting observation worthy of more systematic study; they will look for good scientific evidence.

The scientific method is the best available approach, although it is not without its problems. It starts with observation; a suggestion is made as to what causes what (a hypothesis); the hypothesis is tested in an experiment; if necessary, the hypothesis is modified to account for both the old and new information. The procedure is then repeated until the experimental results no longer require the hypothesis to be changed.

The standard by which medicine establishes whether a treatment has a genuine beneficial effect is the double-blind placebo controlled trial. For example, if you wished to establish that the taking of a vitamin improved behaviour, you would make two types of tablet that were the same colour, size and taste. One would be a dummy tablet, a placebo, while the other would contain the active substance, the vitamin. Randomly, a group of people would be asked to take the tablets without knowing if they were receiving the placebo or the active tablet. It would be important that not only those taking the tablet, but also everybody with whom they interacted, including the scientist testing their behaviour, was unaware of the type of tablet being taken. When neither the subjects nor the scientist knows which tablet is being taken, the study is described as double-blind. If the scientist knows who is taking the active tablets and who is taking the placebos, but the subjects do not, then it is described as a single-blind study. If both the subjects and the scientist know that the former are taking an active tablet, then it is an open trial.

All new drugs are subjected to these types of evaluation. A double-blind study is the only method that excludes the biases of those carrying out the trial. The history of drug evaluation shows that a drug is more likely to be found to improve symptoms when it is examined in an open rather than a single-blind trial, and is more likely to prove beneficial in a single-blind than a double-blind trial. There is no suggestion that anybody is acting in a dishonest manner, but that in poorly designed trials the psychological effects of taking the new 'wonder drug' inevitably produce a large beneficial response. The solution is to ensure an equal psychological response to a dummy pill and to see if the active treatment has additional benefits.

Unfortunately, this type of evidence is rarely available when we are examining the impact of food. Although it is possible to produce a vitamin tablet and a similar placebo, the same approach is difficult, if not impossible, with other aspects of diet. For example, you may wish to examine the influence of decreasing fat in the diet. Obviously, you could not remove foods containing fat from the diet without you and your family being aware of the changes, so the procedure could not be double-blind. In addition, we take so many of our calories in the form of fat that other foods would have to be added to ensure an adequate calorie intake. So if we found a change in behaviour after decreasing fat-intake, we would not know if it was a placebo response and would not be able to distinguish the impact of the removal of the fat from the addition of other foods. These types of problem ensure that it is rarely possible to produce scientific evidence that demonstrates beyond doubt a food-related influence on behaviour.

## Correlations

An alternative approach to the double-blind study, and one that is distinctly second best, is to look for correlations between diet and behaviour. If food additives cause hyperactivity, then you would expect that if you measured the extent to which a group of children were hyperactive and the extent to which they ate food containing additives, then the two measures would correspond. This type of approach is frequently taken, although the results are difficult to interpret.

The problem with the correlational approach is to establish what causes what. Some years ago the birth rate in Copenhagen was found to be associated with the frequency of the sightings of storks. Although such an observation could be quoted by those who propose the theory that storks deliver babies, a scientist would wish to exclude alternative explanations. One such explanation might be that some third factor influences both the human and stork birth-rate. Affluence is one possibility: maybe the Danes have more children at times of economic affluence and at such times they have more spare food to feed the storks, which they happen to like. On the basis of a correlation you cannot definitely conclude that storks deliver babies.

Similarly, if you found that hyperactive children ate more food containing additives it would be difficult to draw precise conclusions on that evidence alone. Certainly, if hyperactivity was caused solely by additives, then you would find that these measures correlated. However, it may be that hyperactivity is not caused by additives but that hyperactivity causes children to eat more food that contain additives. As hyperactive children are impulsive and have difficulty in controlling their behaviour, they may eat more highly processed foods, designed to be attractive to children, that contain high levels of additives. It may be that the correlation reflects a third factor; for example, the behaviour of the parent. If a lack of appropriate parental behaviour causes the child to become hyperactive, and the lack of parental control allows the child to eat what is attractive to children, then a child's behaviour and diet would be related, although one did not cause the other. In fact, the question 'Do additives cause hyperactivity?' is posed in too simple a manner; as always, the answer is complex, and is explored in Chapters 5 and 6.

With all their problems, correlations are valuable. In particular, they suggest new hypotheses, which may be examined more systematically by other means. It is important, however, that their limitations are kept in mind.

## Are we all the same?

The approach of randomly giving half of a group of people a vitamin and the other half a placebo assumes that everybody responds similarly to the vitamin. This assumption might not always be reasonable. For example, people who have a poor diet, and hence low levels of stored vitamins, would be expected to respond beneficially, while people who have a good diet, and hence extensive stores of vitamins, would be expected not to be affected. In addition, there are marked differences in our biology. The amount of vitamin or other nutrient required can differ by several hundred per cent from one individual to another, and the ease with which it is absorbed and the efficiency with which it is stored by the body also differ.

The case study of Clare[13] shows an individual and unusual response to the mineral chromium. In this case a systematic, double-blind investigation was carried out for fourteen months, but there was only one subject, Clare. This procedure which included the giving of placebos allows us to be certain that her problem with headaches responded to chromium. Although it has not been studied, it is extremely unlikely that headaches in most of the population respond to chromium; far better stick to aspirin. If we had correlated chromium intake and the incidence of headaches in a large number of people, it is unlikely that they would have been related. If we had used the double-blind approach with a large number of people, then we would have concluded that chromium was without effect, although such a conclusion ignores the individual need of people like Clare. And although Clare is unusual, she is unlikely to be unique.

### Clare: an unusually high need for chromium

For nearly twenty years Clare had suffered headaches three days out of four. Sometimes they were associated with symptoms of migraine and sometimes they required only an aspirin. At the age of 8 she had been in hospital while tests were run to try to establish the origin of the headaches. They were unsuccessful. Since then she had learned to live with frequent headaches as part of her life. In her mid-20s Clare agreed to take part in an experiment that had nothing to do with headaches and that involved taking a tablet containing various vitamins and minerals. To her surprise, within two days of taking the tablet her headaches stopped. The researcher had been unaware of Clare's problem with headaches and had no explanation for her response.

Over a period of fourteen months various combinations of the vitamins and minerals were taken, as well as placebos, and the incidence of headaches was recorded. The headaches improved when Clare took a chromium supplement, although other vitamins, minerals and a placebo were of no value. She weighed everything that she ate for a week. When her intake of chromium was calculated, it reached recommended levels. It seems that Clare needed a much greater intake of chromium than most of the population. Four years after starting to take chromium Clare's life had been transformed. She had a headache at the most once a month and she had taken up new activities, such as aerobics, which had not been possible previously, as the resulting movement of her head had caused severe headaches.

This kind of systematic study of a single individual is very rare. More typically with case studies, all we have is a report that a vitamin has been given to a single patient in an uncontrolled manner and he or she has recovered. If there is only one patient, can we be sure that he or she is typical of other individuals? Usually, in these cases the patients and the doctors know the treatment that is being offered, so it is unclear whether there is more than a placebo response. As many disorders are subject to spontaneous recovery, especially if there is a psychosomatic element, it is also possible that by chance a treatment will be given at the exact moment when the patient would have recovered without it. If large numbers of patients are given vitamins, by chance alone somebody is going to get better shortly afterwards. If it is the occasion when there is a 'miracle recovery' that we remember and talk about, and we forget the many other patients who did not benefit, then the information is misleading. Very often information from case studies is dismissed for the above reasons, but, like correlations, they are of value to the extent that they suggest ideas that can later be examined systematically.

# CHAPTER 2

# What's Important in Your Diet?

In examining the relationship between aspects of diet and behaviour 'nutrients' are frequently discussed. The food we eat consists of macronutrients – carbohydrate, fat and protein – and micronutrients – vitamins and minerals.

## *Macronutrients*

### Carbohydrates

Food contains three major groups of carbohydrates: sugars, starches, and cellulose and related materials. Sugars and starches are the major sources of energy. The attractive sweet taste of sugars means that they are widely used in food preparation, and their ability to act as a preservative is particularly valuable.

Starches consist of long chains of units of glucose, a simple sugar. They are indigestible if eaten raw in foods such as potatoes or flour, but change into a form that can be digested when heated in the presence of water.

Cellulose also consists of long chains of units of simple sugars, but is indigestible by humans. It is the major component of dietary fibre in fruit and vegetables. There has been considerable interest in the possibility that a tendency to eat carbohydrate may reflect an attempt to improve mood by people who are depressed (see Chapter 11), and that a diet containing too much sugar can have adverse consequences (see Chapter 7).

## Fats

Fat makes an important contribution to the taste and texture of many foods, and a diet devoid of fat would be unpleasant to eat. Fats offer a more concentrated source of energy than carbohydrates and are the form in which the energy reserves of many animals are stored. They can be visible or invisible. Visible fats include butter, margarine and the fat on meat that we can see. Invisible fats are hidden inside foods such as milk, lean meat, cakes and biscuits. Chemically, fats consist mainly of a mixture of triglycerides, each of which is a combination of three fatty acids and a unit of glycerol. The differences between one fat or oil and another are a reflection of differences in fatty acids.

There are dozens of different fatty acids, which are classified as one of two types. Saturated fatty acids are the major constituents of hard fats such as lard. Unsaturated fatty acids are found in all fats but in high amounts in olive and other vegetable oils. The body has the capability to manufacture most fatty acids, but there are a few, such as linoleic, linolenic and arachidonic acids, it cannot make. Because the body needs them and cannot make them, they have to form part of the diet. They are therefore called essential fatty acids. The importance of an adequate intake of essential fatty acids in brain development is discussed in Chapter 3.

As high levels of cholesterol in the blood are associated with an increased risk of coronary heart disease, and a high intake of saturated fats increases cholesterol levels, it is recommended that the intake of fat, particularly saturated fat, is decreased. The psychological consequences of attempting to decrease fat intake are considered in Chapter 11.

## Proteins

Proteins consist of chains of hundreds of amino acids. There are about twenty amino acids combined in a multitude of different sequences. The essential amino acids, which have to be present in the diet, can be distinguished from the non-essential amino acids, which can be manufactured by the body. A lack of protein during critical stages in the brain's development can cause lasting problems (see Chapter 3).

Most animal protein is similar to that found in humans in terms of the amino acids it provides. In contrast, a single vegetable protein differs from the protein needed by humans in terms of the amino acids it provides. For this reason a vegetarian meal needs a variety of food items to ensure that all amino acids are supplied in adequate quantities. The nutritional advantage of animal foods over vegetables is, however, more in the provision of other nutrients, such as vitamin $B_{12}$, iron and vitamin D, rather than the quality of the protein.

## Micronutrients

### Vitamins

At the beginning of the twentieth century it became apparent that we need more than protein, fats and carbohydrate in our diet. These additional nutrients, which are needed in only small amounts, were originally called 'vital amines' in the knowledge that they were vital for life and the mistaken belief that they were all chemicals known as amines. The term was later contracted to vitamins. Although all the roles played by vitamins in the body are not fully understood, we know that vitamins have many important functions (Figure 2.1).

There are two broad groups of vitamins, those that are water soluble and those that are fat soluble. Many foods contain both fat- and water-based constituents, and therefore may contain both fat- and water-soluble vitamins. For example, cauliflower, bacon and beef all contain thiamine, riboflavin and other water-soluble vitamins as well as vitamin E, which is fat soluble. If the diet offers inadequate levels of a vitamin, a deficiency disease may result; for example, the disease scurvy is the result of an insufficient amount of vitamin C, and pellagra is a result of too little niacin. Often before a deficiency disease is apparent, a low intake can produce symptoms of a psychological nature. Table 2.1 lists some common vitamins, some foods in which they are found and psychological problems associated with deficiency. It should not, however, be assumed that

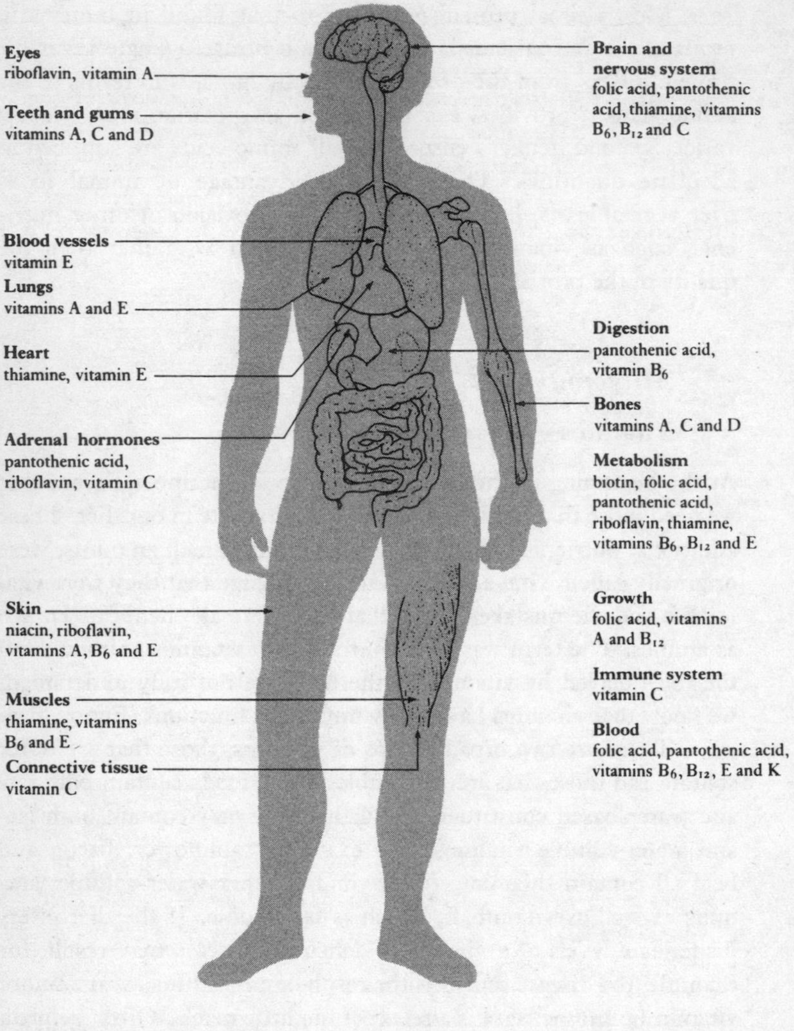

**Eyes**
riboflavin, vitamin A

**Teeth and gums**
vitamins A, C and D

**Blood vessels**
vitamin E

**Lungs**
vitamins A and E

**Heart**
thiamine, vitamin E

**Adrenal hormones**
pantothenic acid,
riboflavin, vitamin C

**Skin**
niacin, riboflavin,
vitamins A, $B_6$ and E

**Muscles**
thiamine, vitamins
$B_6$ and E

**Connective tissue**
vitamin C

**Brain and
nervous system**
folic acid, pantothenic
acid, thiamine, vitamins
$B_6$, $B_{12}$ and C

**Digestion**
pantothenic acid,
vitamin $B_6$

**Bones**
vitamins A, C and D

**Metabolism**
biotin, folic acid,
pantothenic acid,
riboflavin, thiamine,
vitamins $B_6$, $B_{12}$ and E

**Growth**
folic acid, vitamins
A and $B_{12}$

**Immune system**
vitamin C

**Blood**
folic acid, pantothenic acid,
vitamins $B_6$, $B_{12}$, E and K

*Figure 2.1* **Primary functions of vitamins**
Most vitamins have a number of roles in the body, many associated with
enzymes, the proteins that are responsible for chemical reactions.

*Table 2.1* **Vitamins that in low supply may cause psychological problems**

| Vitamins | Foods containing high levels | Symptoms of deficiency* |
| --- | --- | --- |
| Folic acid | Offal, raw green leafy vegetables | Tiredness, mild depression, confusion |
| Niacin | Meats, cheese, fish, eggs | Emotional instability, sleep and memory problems |
| Riboflavin | Milk, cheese, eggs, kidney, liver | Depression, lethargy |
| Thiamine | Milk, pork, eggs, whole-grain cereals | Memory problems, irritability, fatigue |
| Vitamin $B_6$ | Meats, fish, eggs, cereals, some vegetables | Fatigue, irritability, insomnia |
| Vitamin $B_{12}$ | Liver, eggs, cheese, meat, fish | Memory impairment, mild depression, fear |
| Vitamin C | Fruit, vegetables | Fatigue, depression, hysteria |

\* Vitamin deficiencies are never the only possible cause of these problems and are in practice uncommon.

vitamin deficiencies are a common cause of psychological problems or that the same symptoms cannot result for other reasons. The possibility that either a low vitamin intake or supplements that provide levels in excess of those provided by the diet can influence both mood and the way people think has been considered extensively (see Chapters 4, 9 and 11).

### Minerals

About fifteen minerals are known to be essential for life and must be obtained from food. A minute amount of another five minerals is necessary, and it is difficult to imagine any diet without an adequate supply. Those needed in relatively large amounts are termed the major minerals whereas others, needed in much smaller quantities, are called trace elements. Table 2.2 lists some of these

*Table 2.2* **Some major and trace minerals**

| Major minerals | Foods containing high levels | Function | Symptoms of deficiency |
|---|---|---|---|
| Calcium | Milk, cheese, bread | Bones, teeth | Rickets, osteoporosis |
| Iron | Meat, offal, eggs | Use of oxygen; found in brain | Anaemia, fatigue |
| Magnesium | Vegetables, but widespread | Energy liberation | Rare |
| Phosphorus | Most foods | Bones, energy liberation | Unknown |
| *Trace elements* | | | |
| Chromium | Widespread | Use of glucose | See Clare's case study |
| Iodine | Milk, meat, eggs | Thyroid hormones | Goitre, learning disorders |
| Selenium | Meat, cereals | Red blood cell enzyme | Heart problems, depressed mood |
| Zinc | Widespread | Many enzymes, wound healing | Poor appetite, lethargy, irritability |

essential minerals. A low intake of iron is a common cause of problems (see Chapter 11).

## *Judging your diet*

How can we tell if we are well fed? The simple answer is that we cannot. Not even the most well-qualified nutritionists can say whether we are, or are not, well nourished. They may think it highly likely that we are well fed, but there is no way that they can know for certain. This assertion may seem unlikely, as the side of many breakfast cereal packages will tell us that one serving will provide sufficient of a particular vitamin to give us a third of the recommended daily amount. It is, however, important to understand the meaning of a recommended daily amount, or RDA.

The committee that drew up the American RDAs defined them as 'the levels of intake of essential nutrients that, on the basis of scientific knowledge, are judged by the Food and Nutrition Board to be adequate to meet the known nutritional needs of practically all healthy persons'.[1] Such a definition sounds fine, but its true meaning is hidden by the use of the word 'needs' – what is being discussed? The United Kingdom committee charged with the same task defined what it meant by 'needs'.

Classically, the requirement of an individual for a nutrient has been the amount required to prevent clinical signs of deficiency ... it can be argued that societies should expect more than the basic need to avoid deficiency, to allow for periods of low intake or high demand ... Claims have also been made that at very high levels of intake some nutrients have especially beneficial or therapeutic effects but the panel decided that these effects did not fall within their definition of requirement.[2]

'Need' can mean many things: the avoiding of a deficiency disease, the maintaining of adequate stores of vitamins and minerals or the achieving of optimal functioning. It is clearly stated that the RDAs are intended to achieve lower rather than higher objectives, although in building in a safety margin many would argue that they may achieve more than their limited objectives. Some of the many factors that influence our need for vitamins and minerals are:

- alcohol consumption
- bioavailability of nutrients
- biological individuality
- climate
- composition of diet
- disease or metabolic disorders
- medication
- physical activity
- smoking

The important point is that we differ markedly in our need for micronutrients; an intake that is adequate for one person may not be adequate for another. The need for a vitamin may differ by as much as several hundred per cent from one individual to another,[3] a reflection of basic differences in our biology and lifestyle. The RDA is therefore defined as a level of intake that will satisfy the needs of 95 per cent of the population. It follows that there are many in the population who are healthy if they consume less than the RDA.

What is very clear is that the RDAs were never intended to ensure that optimal psychological functioning could be achieved. The measures against which the adequacy of vitamin intake are assessed are biological rather than psychological in nature. Perhaps psychological measures should be used, as with many vitamins the first signs of deficiency are psychological; people may feel a little depressed, irritable or even paranoid.[4]

Whatever their objectives, how much faith can we place in these RDAs? The comments about the RDAs made by a British professor of nutrition, who had sat on one of the committees that established them, are illuminating.

The answer 'We do not know' was not acceptable . . . so a best guess was made.

I can confirm that no self-respecting scientist could derive any professional satisfaction from those miserable little pamphlets.

. . . the frailty of their scientific basis was all too easily revealed.

For another 30 nutrients the scientists' answer 'We do not know' was perforce accepted.[5]

These comments, published in the *British Medical Journal*, are considerably more colourful than those normally expected from a professor talking about his subject. However, they say little with which a well-trained nutritionist would not agree, although probably in more measured terms. It is not appropriate to list the many problems associated with the calculation of the RDAs, but the above comments illustrate the widespread acceptance that their scientific basis is insecure. As confirmation of this view the British committee dealing with this matter noted: 'For most nutrients the panel found insufficient data to establish any of these Dietary Reference Values (RDA) with great confidence. There are inherent errors . . .'[6]

Nutrition is far from an exact science. As the RDA is the standard against which dietary intake is compared, it is clear that little, if anything, can be said with certainty. The RDAs are, however, the best standards we have and should be accepted for what they are: an honest attempt at performing an impossible task. They are as much legal and political necessities as scientifically valid statements. If the law says that when breakfast cereals are manufactured and a vitamin is added, the manufacturer must express the amount added as a percentage of the RDA, then somebody has to define the RDA. The nutritionist is necessarily given the task, although the information needed is often fragmentary and the figure produced of doubtful validity.

## What surveys tell us

If diet is going to influence behaviour, then it is more likely to be demonstrated in those people who consume a poor diet and have less than optimal stores of various nutrients. It follows that the repeated assurance of government scientists that our diet is adequate, if true, makes it less likely that our psychological functioning is influenced by diet. But is it the case that diet in industrialized societies is uniformly good? In 1988 in the United States the Surgeon General's Report on Nutrition and Health recognized that the most prevalent nutritional problems among Americans were due to overeating and imbalances in dietary intake rather than deficiencies of a single nutrient: diets were too high in fat, calories, salt and alcohol, and too low in fibre. It was recommended that people eat more wholegrain foods, cereal products, fruit and vegetables.[7]

In fact, the assumption that there are no deficiencies of single nutrients may not be valid. For example, in France when blood levels of apparently healthy children were examined for their vitamin A and E content, 5 per cent were found to be at risk of deficiency.[8]

In Britain one of the first decisions of Margaret Thatcher's Government was to pass the 1980 Education Act, which meant that local authorities no longer had to provide a midday school meal; if they did, it did not have to meet any minimum nutritional standards. Naturally, there was great concern that children in the poorest section of society were being deprived of the only adequate meal that they ate. Several years previously, when she had been Minster of Education, Margaret Thatcher had removed the provision of free school milk, a decision that was condemned by many nutritionists who saw milk as an important source of calcium and that earned Mrs Thatcher one of her many political nicknames, 'Milk snatcher Thatcher'.

Part of the attempt to diffuse the political opposition to these measures was the promise that the nutritional consequences would be monitored. The result was a survey of 2,697 schoolchildren, who weighed everything they ate for one week in 1983. When the full survey was eventually published in 1989, the Minister of Health, David Mellor, told the press, 'This is a highly detailed scientific analysis ... It shows that schoolchildren in all social classes were well nourished and thriving ... All of them had adequate, or more than adequate intakes of nutrients.'[9]

This reassuring conclusion was politically and economically convenient for the government, who, having devalued the nutritional importance of school meals and removed school milk, needed the diet of children to be given a clean bill of health. Why, if the conclusions were really so politically convenient, was there a reluctance to publish the findings?

An early draft of the report was circulated in time for the government committee dealing with the survey that met in December 1984. A complete draft was available for their meeting in April 1985.[10] By early 1986, according to responses to parliamentary questions, its publication had been put off three times. The *Daily Telegraph* reported:

A so-far unpublished report commissioned by the Government from its nutritional advisors at the Department of Health shows that Britain's overweight teenagers are consuming masses of fatty and sugary foods. Independent dietetians say the report shows that children are storing up future health problems by eating the wrong food in their developing years but the report is noticeably silent on the possible consequences of teenagers' high fat, high sugar and low fibre choice of food.[11]

A week later a press release announced the publication of a preliminary report in which Ray Whitney, then junior Health Minister, said, 'The preliminary results are encouraging and show that our children enjoy adequate nutrition.'

On 14 April 1986 Granada Television broadcast a special programme entitled 'The Threatened Generation', based on the findings of the survey *The Diets of British Schoolchildren*.[12] In that programme Professor John Garrow said:

The proportion of obese children is increasing, and that is worrying, because the evidence is that the younger you become obese and the longer you have been obese the more likely you are to develop diabetes and high blood pressure.[13]

In the same programme Dr Cummings of the Dunn Clinical Nutrition Centre at Cambridge commented:

This report shows quite clearly that the diet these children are eating, if we are to believe current nutritional guidelines, is likely to leave them open to developing heart disease and cancer ... This is the sort of diet that has been condemned ... as the one likely to lead in later life to a whole variety of ill-health.[14]

When the government wishes to survey the country's diet, it naturally uses the RDA as the bench-mark against which to measure our nutrition. There are no other standards against which the diets of British schoolchildren could be compared. There is a rule of thumb: if the average intake of a vitamin is above the RDA, then the diet is adequate. However, by the nature of such calculations, many people will have an intake below the average. An extreme example would be a situation where half of us had none of a vitamin in our diet and the other half of the population had twice the RDA. In this totally improbable case the average level of consumption would be the RDA, and if we used the rule of thumb uncritically, we would conclude that the intake of this vitamin was adequate. Clearly, such a conclusion would be unreasonable, and would not be drawn. Those of us with no vitamin in our diet would suffer from a deficiency disorder and eventual death. It is obvious that you should look at the lowest intakes before concluding that there are no members of the community whose diet is inadequate. We should not overlook the low vitamin intake of even a few in the population just because the intake of the majority is adequate.

The conclusion that all British children are well nourished, thriving and have an adequate intake of nutrients relied on the crude rule of thumb that if the average intake is above the RDA then there is unlikely to be a problem. There is another rule of thumb that could have been used but was not.

If you consume 100 per cent of the RDA, then it is unlikely that you will have a problem. If you consume 0 per cent of the RDA, then you definitely will have a problem. As the intake declines from 100 to 0 per cent, the probability increases that you will have a problem. Traditionally, nutritionists have suggested that an intake less than 70 per cent of the RDA gives grounds for concern. If the intake is even less, then the concern is that much greater.

Table 2.3 reports the percentage of British schoolchildren whose diet was found to offer less than 70 and less than 50 per cent of the RDA of a number of vitamins. Although the survey found many children were well fed, it gave grounds for concern about the vitamin intake of others. That some children had a very low vitamin intake does not allow the conclusion that they necessarily have a problem, but that possibility should have been considered.

A more accurate method of assessing whether the diet offers sufficient quantities of vitamins is to take blood samples and measure vitamin levels using biochemical tests. Table 2.4 lists the results of such tests on a group of 243 young, apparently healthy British adults. The picture is similar to that in the study of children's diet: although many of the subjects have levels of vitamins that are satisfactory, the levels of a minority were marginal or even low enough to be described as deficient.

*Table 2.3* Percentage of children with a low intake of various micronutrients

| | Boys | | | | Girls | | | |
|---|---|---|---|---|---|---|---|---|
| | 10–11 years | | 14–15 years | | 10–11 years | | 14–15 years | |
| | <70% RDA | <50% RDA | <70% RDA | <50% RDA | <70% RDA | <50% RDA | <70% RDA | <50% RDA |
| Calcium | 9 | 3 | 5 | 2 | 17 | 5 | 11 | 4 |
| Iron | 25 | 2 | 13 | 1 | 50 | 8 | 36 | 10 |
| Nicotinic acid | 0 | 0 | 0 | 0 | 0 | 0 | 0 | 0 |
| Riboflavin | 7 | 2 | 10 | 5 | 12 | 4 | 25 | 11 |
| Thiamine | 5 | 1 | 8 | 3 | 6 | 2 | 9 | 3 |
| Vitamin A | 17 | 11 | 34 | 28 | 33 | 26 | 34 | 22 |
| Vitamin B₆* | 61 | 19 | 59 | 11 | 80 | 32 | 75 | 20 |

* US RDA

*Source:* Data from Subcommittee on Nutritional Surveillance, *The Diets of British Schoolchildren*, London, HMSO, 1989.

*Table 2.4* **Vitamin status of young British adults**

|  | Male (%) | | | Female (%) | | |
|---|---|---|---|---|---|---|
|  | Deficient | Marginal | Adequate | Deficient | Marginal | Adequate |
| Folic acid | 0 | 5 | 95 | 0 | 7 | 93 |
| Riboflavin | 20 | 17 | 63 | 29 | 28 | 43 |
| Thiamine | 5 | 17 | 78 | 2 | 18 | 80 |
| Vitamin A | 0 | 2 | 98 | 0 | 18 | 82 |
| Vitamin B$_6$ | 28 | 15 | 57 | 36 | 27 | 37 |
| Vitamin B$_{12}$ | 1 | 2 | 97 | 2 | 3 | 95 |
| Vitamin E | 0 | 1 | 99 | 0 | 0 | 100 |

*Source:* D. Benton, J. Haller and J. Fordy, 'The vitamin status of a sample of young British adults', submitted for publication.

## Prospect

So far basic information about diet and its measurement has been discussed as background for the coming chapters, which examine attempts to relate the intake of both macro- and micronutrients to psychological functioning. It would be reasonable to suggest that only a poor diet will adversely influence the way we think; by definition, a good diet can cause no adverse effects. For anyone taking such a view, evidence from nutritional surveys that people universally consume an adequate diet would strongly suggest that psychological functioning is not influenced by diet.

When considering the possibility that the intelligence of school-children might be enhanced by taking vitamin and mineral supplements, Professor Naismith, of King's College London, commented, 'I would be surprised if mental ability could be affected by diet . . . in my opinion the majority of school children nowadays are well nourished.'[15] His predecessor, Professor Yudkin, said the same thing in a more pithy way, which vividly illustrates the certainty of nutritionists that children's diets are not short of vitamins: 'Ludicrous meaningless nonsense'.[16]

For these two professors of nutrition the survey of the diets of British schoolchildren, discussed above, was sufficient to dismiss as unlikely the finding that some children respond to vitamin supplementation. However, as we saw in Table 2.3, the survey found that a minority of children had low intakes of some vitamins and minerals; we should consider that at least these children may be influenced by supplementation (see Chapter 4).

It may appear that the survey of the diets of British schoolchildren and similar surveys demonstrate that diet is on occasion inadequate, and thus that behaviour can be influenced adversely. Such a conclusion is not justified. In fact, nutritional surveys tell us little that is relevant to the question 'Does diet influence us psychologically?' – indeed, they were never intended to, and we must look elsewhere, to psychological rather than nutritional research, for the answers.

To use the RDA as the bench-mark against which to measure the adequacy of diet is to use a measure that was never designed to achieve either optimal functioning in general, or optimal psychological functioning in particular. That there are grounds for concern about someone's diet is not the same as saying that there is definitely a problem. We should wipe the slate clean and dismiss the sweeping generalizations that diet is adequate, if not good. Such a view may be right or it may be wrong; we will find out only by the use of well-designed scientific studies.

It is to be hoped that the reader starts with an open mind about whether diet does or does not influence behaviour. The evidence needs to be examined in a sober manner. Attempts to scientifically study the impact of diet on behaviour, limited although they are, will be outlined. Rarely, if ever, are there simple answers. It should be remembered that diet is only one of many factors that influence human behaviour, and in most of us its influence rarely predominates. However, there is a small proportion of the population who respond to their diet in a dramatic way.

# CHAPTER 3

# Early Influences

The young of all mammals, particularly humans, have large heads compared with the size of their body. This is because the brain develops more rapidly than the rest of the body. Figure 3.1 shows that the increase in weight of the human brain occurs most rapidly in the last third of pregnancy and the first year of life. At birth the baby's total weight is about 5 per cent of an adult's, yet the brain has already reached 25 per cent of its adult weight. At the end of the first year of life 90–95 per cent of the adult number of brain cells are present.[1] Obviously, the rapidly growing brain requires a good source of nutrition, and it is reasonable to ask if malnutrition during this period will have long-term implications. In other words, will a poor diet during this critical period of growth cause problems in the brain's development that cannot be solved later if the diet improves?

From the study of animals scientists have been able to distinguish the various aspects of the brain that develop at this time. The neurones, the brain cells that pass electrical messages, are formed; the neurones become covered with a fatty sheath that acts as an insulator; a large number of connections between neurones develop, which allows a rich variety of messages to be processed. Undernutrition during the spurt in brain growth results not in a smaller number of neurones, but rather in fewer connections between them. Undernutrition before or after this time does not have the same effect, nor does a subsequently good diet enable the neurones to develop these connections later.[2] A poor diet does not damage the brain, but rather prevents normal development in the first place.

Scientists also know from the study of animals that malnutrition and an unstimulating environment have very similar conse-

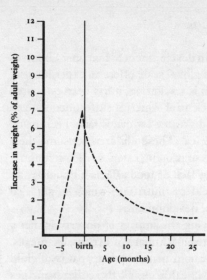

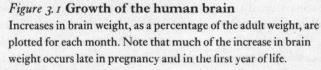

*Figure 3.1* **Growth of the human brain**
Increases in brain weight, as a percentage of the adult weight, are
plotted for each month. Note that much of the increase in brain
weight occurs late in pregnancy and in the first year of life.

quences. The type of study on which this conclusion is based
involves raising laboratory rats in either an impoverished or an
enriched environment. An impoverished environment is a standard
cage with a good supply of food, water and bedding. An enriched
environment is one that in addition contains a series of ladders,
wheels and objects to explore. Rats in an impoverished environment
are similar to those who were malnourished during the critical stage
of brain development: their brains have fewer connections between
the cells. In animals we can be certain not only that early malnutrition causes permanent changes in brain structure, but also that the
impact of undernutrition can be ameliorated by environmental stimulation; that is, environmental stimulation results in the development
of more connections between neurones. Nutrition does not act in
isolation from other environmental events; this conclusion also applies to humans.

## Malnutrition in humans

Does malnutrition influence brain development in humans? Unfortunately, human malnutrition on a global scale offers an experiment of nature. The scale of the problem is staggering; it has been estimated that 24 per cent of children in Central America suffer moderate or severe malnutrition;[3] similar and greater estimates have been made in Africa, Asia and South America. These children consume diets that provide inadequate amounts of protein, calories and micronutrients. Although a life-threatening lack of food afflicts a minority, an even greater number suffer mild malnutrition, which might also have implications for intellectual development.

A major problem in studying the impact of poverty is that a lack of food is typically associated with many other disadvantages: disease, infestation, lack of education, poor housing, apathy of child and parents, a mother with poor health. As all these disadvantages have the potential to impair cognitive development, it is impossible to isolate the impact of malnutrition.

The study of severe malnutrition brings additional problems. The conditions associated with malnutrition in non-industrialized countries do not allow the accurate monitoring of diet, certainly not for prolonged periods. Given that a very poor diet will be deficient in virtually every aspect of nutrition, it is impossible to establish which nutrients are critical. If malnutrition lasts a lifetime, how can the stage at which it has its impact be established? How do we know at which aspects of mood, personality or intellectual functioning we should look?

### Retrospective studies

In retrospective studies a group of children known to have suffered in the past from gross malnutrition are compared with a group who have not. A review of the many studies of this nature concluded, 'They strongly suggest that early malnutrition has long-term and adverse consequences for social and emotional development with attention, social responsiveness and emotional adjustment significantly affected.'[4] However, a poor diet is typically only one of many problems, and its relative importance cannot be established using this type of approach. Perhaps a safer conclusion is that there are long-term consequences of growing up in grossly underprivileged conditions.

## Prospective studies

Given that retrospective studies of malnutrition give data that are impossible to interpret, prospective studies are of more interest. In prospective studies children are given food supplements and their progress is compared with that of similar children who do not receive supplementation.

In one study poor Mexican mothers were given a nutritionally adequate diet from early pregnancy to the third month after birth. Their children scored more highly on a series of achievement tests in primary school than did other children.[5] Although an improved diet may have been important, the children acquired prestige within the community and that may also have played a role. The idea that diet does not act in isolation is supported by the finding that children in Bogotá who were given a combination of tutoring and nutritional supplementation benefited more than those who received only food.[6]

In another study children in Taiwan whose mothers were given a high-calorie and protein supplement during pregnancy and breast-feeding, had enhanced motor, but not mental, scores at the age of 8 months.[7] That motor development is particularly sensitive to supplementation is a common finding, in animals as well as humans, and may reflect the rapid development of the cerebellum, an area of the brain important in the control of motor activity.

There is a consistent impression from the growing number of prospective studies that 'long-standing energy deficit has detrimental effects not only on growth, but on the child's cognitive development'.[8]

Although the consistency of the findings is gratifying, it should not be assumed that the effects are necessarily large or long-term. In the study of children in Colombia[9] those who received food supplements only for the first six months of life no longer demonstrated developmental benefits at the age of 3 years.

One way of attempting to establish the role of diet is to examine children in industrialized societies who have the advantages of that society but suffer malnutrition because they are unable to adequately absorb or metabolize food. It is hoped that the impact of malnutrition can thus be distinguished from other disadvantages. A study in the United States reported that the social and emotional nature of children hospitalized with bowel problems was not different from those not having these problems.[10] Although intelligence scores were not different, these children had a higher rate of school failure. In this situation early malnutrition was associated with a socially privileged environment and the consequences were much smaller than those found in non-industrialized countries. It is unclear to what extent the school failure reflected malnutrition rather than being ill.

### Dutch hunger winter

Important information about the impact of nutrition while the baby is still in the womb is still being gained from studies of people born in the Netherlands in 1945.[11]

On 17 September 1944 Allied paratroopers landed at Arnhem in an attempt to capture a bridge that would have allowed their troops to rapidly cross the Rhine, an operation commemorated in the film *A Bridge Too Far*. At the same time the Dutch government-in-exile in London called on Dutch rail workers to strike. The paratroopers were unsuccessful, and as a reprisal the Nazis imposed a transport embargo in October 1944 that lasted until liberation in May 1945. Cities in the west of the Netherlands, including Amsterdam, The Hague, Rotterdam and Utrecht, received little food for six months. Figure 3.2 shows the area affected.

A famine resulted. Never before had a severe famine taken place for a prescribed period, in a precise area, where the degree of famine was known. At the most, 1,000 calories a day were consumed, typically less, and these came mainly from bread and

*Figure 3.2* **Dutch hunger winter**

During the Second World War people living in the cities marked with a circle suffered famine; those in cities marked with a triangle have been used for comparison.

*Source:* Z. A. Stein, M. W. Susser, G. Saenger and F. Marolla, *Famine and Human Development: the Dutch Hunger Winter of 1944/45*, Oxford, OUP, 1975.

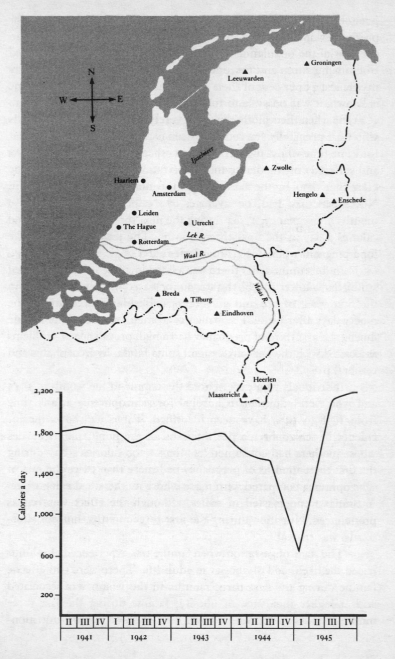

potatoes. From the beginning of the famine special rations for pregnant women were stopped. The famine was so severe that 10 per cent of the population suffered hunger oedema, thousands died from malnutrition and there was a sharp decrease in fertility. Many people lost 25 per cent of their weight. As the duration of the famine is known, it was possible to follow up those who were in the womb at a time when their mothers were severely short of food. Individuals who were prenatally starved have been compared with those born at the same time whose mothers lived in other areas of the Netherlands and suffered only moderate food deprivation; that is, they had 1,500 calories a day. In the famine area the mothers of those born in November 1945 had, on average, 672 calories in the first three months of pregnancy, 1,762 during the next three months and 2,090 calories a day in the final three months. The recommended intake for a pregnant woman is 2,140 calories a day.

In the famine areas there was a large increase in the number of stillbirths, a lower live birth rate, an increased incidence of death in the first week of life and an increased likelihood of death in the ninety days after birth. The babies of women exposed to the famine during the first third of pregnancy had a high prevalence of problems associated with the nervous system: spina bifida, hydrocephalus and cerebral palsy.

Individuals who experienced the famine in the womb in 1945 and who were admitted to hospital for schizophrenia at any time from 1978 to 1989 have been identified. Table 3.1 shows the incidence of schizophrenia per thousand of the population. Females whose mothers had consumed less than 1,000 calories a day during the first three months of pregnancy had more than twice the rate of schizophrenia compared with those whose mothers had eaten more. A similar trend existed in males, although the effect was not as pronounced. Nutrition during the first three months, but not afterwards, was critical.

The stage of gestation when famine was experienced also influenced the likelihood of obesity in adult life. There were two effects: famine during the first three months in the womb was associated with a higher incidence of obesity; famine during the last three months was associated with a lower level of obesity. Some nutrition-

*Table 3.1* **Diet in first three months of pregnancy and schizophrenia in offspring**

| Schizophrenia per thousand of population | Mother's intake of calories while pregnant | | |
| --- | --- | --- | --- |
| | Over 1,500 | 1,000–1,500 | Less than 1,000 |
| Males | 1.4 | 1.3 | 2.0 |
| Females | 1.1 | 1.1 | 2.8 |

*Source:* Data from E. S. Susser, P. H. Shang and P. Lin, 'Schizophrenia after prenatal exposure to the Dutch Hunger Winter of 1944–1945', *Archives of General Psychiatry*, 49, 1992, 983–8.

ists speculate that the adequacy of nutrition may have influenced the development of those areas of the brain that control food intake.

In the Netherlands all males join the army for national service at the age of 19 and at this time take intelligence tests. The Dutch famine allowed the examination of the idea that intelligence will be less if the brain is malnourished at the stage of maximum growth. The IQs of those who at the time of the famine had been in the womb of a severely starved mother were not significantly different from those whose mothers had lived in other areas of the Netherlands at this time.[12]

These data are sometimes quoted as demonstrating that prenatal nutrition does not influence intellectual development. However, in this wartime condition the comparison is between a poor diet and a very poor diet, and both groups may have suffered. The famine was also relatively short-lived, and the child may have benefited from the mother's store of nutrients. It may be that all that was demonstrated is that when it comes to nutrition, the foetus rather than the mother is given preference.

The data from the Dutch famine are interesting, but as it was an experiment of nature, and not a laboratory study, there are problems of interpretation. The winter of 1944/5 was cold and fuel was scarce; disease was common, including tuberculosis, dysentery and typhoid. Many unusual items – for example, tulip bulbs – were eaten. A friend who was a child in Rotterdam during the famine tells how her father, almost without the strength to get out of bed, went to the local stream to catch sticklebacks that he ate whole, including the spines. It is difficult to exclude the possibility that a toxic food was eaten in the search for calories. Alternatively, a poor diet may have increased the incidence of a particular disease that, in turn, may have predisposed individuals to schizophrenia.

Beyond noting that severe famine in the first three months of pregnancy is associated in an increased incidence of schizophrenia it is difficult to draw conclusions. In industrialized societies such extremes of malnutrition in pregnant women occur rarely, if at all. It is unclear what was missing from the diet that led to and increased the likelihood of schizophrenia. If the problem was an extremely low intake of calories, then the finding has little relevance for Western societies today. If the important factor was a low intake of a specific vitamin or mineral, then it may have significance in some countries or sections of a population. We simply do not know what aspect of diet is important. As women were more influenced by their mother's diet than men, it may be that schizophrenia is a syndrome with several causes, with women being more vulnerable to diet than men.

## Protein–energy supplementation in industrialized societies

There have been very few attempts to examine the impact of supplementing the diet of poor people in industrialized societies. In one study poor pregnant women in New York were given protein–energy supplements: these offered either 6 g or 40 g of protein a day, together with a range of vitamins and minerals.[13] Supplementation during pregnancy resulted in an increased length of gestation and a decreased number of low-birth-weight infants, particularly if the mother smoked. It was also associated with improvement on two measures of visual perception and longer bouts of play when the children were 1 year old. There was also evidence, however, that 40 g of protein could be associated with a higher number of premature births and hence neonatal deaths. It cannot necessarily be assumed that if a small nutritional supplement is beneficial, a larger supplement will bring additional benefits or any benefit at all.

In Louisiana low-income mothers in the last third of pregnancy, and their children in the first year of life, were supplied with a range of foods such as eggs and milk.[14] When compared at the age of 5 those children who had received the additional food had enhanced intellectual, attentional and motor performances, and higher school grades. Performance was better when supplementation began before the first year of age, after which the brain's growth spurt has largely finished.

A related question is whether the nature of an artificial milk influences the behaviour of the child. It does, at least in premature children.

In one of an excellent series of studies of the impact of diet on development, Alan Lucas and his colleagues at the University of Cambridge randomly gave low-birth-weight infants either a standard cow's-milk-based formula or a special pre-term baby's formula that contained 40 per cent more protein, 18 per cent more energy and a wide range of vitamins and minerals. The period of this feeding began at birth and lasted thirty days. Figure 3.3 shows that at 18 months the development of the infants who had received the enriched formula was more advanced than that of those who had been fed with the standard formulation. At 18 months those who had received the enriched formula 'had major developmental advantages, more so in motor than mental function: the advantages were striking in small-for-gestational-age infants and in males'.[15] The formula improved motor development in particular. However, both social and mental development, and specifically language, were also advanced.

It is unclear whether the type of baby food consumed would similarly influence the development of children who were not born early. A premature baby is born with a brain at an earlier stage of development, and it is possible that the nature of the diet is more critical at some stages of brain development than at others. Certainly, the effects of diet were particularly powerful in infants who were very small at birth.

There are very few studies of the impact of improving the

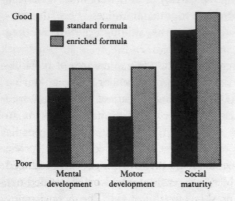

*Figure 3.3* **Baby-milk influences development**
Infants were randomly given either traditional baby milk or one
enriched with protein and vitamins and minerals. At 18 months the
motor development of those having had the enriched formula at
birth was significantly advanced.
*Source:* Data from A. Lucas *et al.*, *Lancet*, 335, 1990, 1477–81.

diet of poor mothers and young children in industrialized countries,
so firm conclusions cannot as yet be drawn. How extensive are any
problems? What in the diet is important? What is the nature of any
benefits and for how long do they last? There is an urgent need to
examine the association between poverty, low birth-weight children
and the possibility that improved nutrition may prove psychologically beneficial.

### Perinatal vitamin–mineral supplementation

Most studies of supplementation have given a range of foods that
increase the amount of protein in the diet; vitamins and minerals
by themselves have been administered less frequently. In a study
carried out in the 1930s in the United States the development of
normal babies who were supplied with milk fortified with B
vitamins was contrasted with those given non-fortified milk. At 6

months the infants receiving the extra vitamins were more advanced on fifty-nine out of sixty-five developmental indices. This superiority was still apparent at 9 and 12 months, although the controls had partially caught up.[16]

Pregnant women attending a clinic in a slum area of Norfolk, Virginia, were given either vitamin supplements or a placebo during pregnancy and lactation.[17] Both at 3 and 4 years of age the children who had received the vitamins scored significantly better on an intelligence test. However, a group of Kentucky mountain people did not respond similarly. The difference may reflect dietary factors: the Kentucky mountain people raised their own meat and produced their own fruit and vegetables, whereas those in Norfolk tended not to have gardens and relied on shops for their food. The inconsistency of the findings illustrates the difficulty in drawing general conclusions and assuming that a similar response will be obtained in different sections of the population. Without any detailed measure of the dietary status, and other characteristics of these two groups, it has been impossible to establish the factors that produce a positive response to vitamin supplementation.

### Spina bifida

The Dutch famine was associated with an increased incidence of abnormalities of the nervous system, including spina bifida, a neural tube disorder in which the developing spinal cord is left exposed because the bones and other surrounding tissues do not develop correctly. More recent research has confirmed the importance of diet in the development of the nervous system. In particular, it has been established that folic acid, one of the B vitamins, has a role in preventing spina bifida and other neural tube disorders.

In early studies women who had already had a child with spina bifida were given vitamin supplements, in particular folic acid. The likelihood of having a second child with spina bifida decreased to about one-seventh of the rate of similar women who had not taken the vitamin.[18] This was not a double-blind placebo controlled study; the mothers could choose whether or not they took the vitamin, and if they did, they were compared with mothers who chose not to. Did this uncontrolled approach mean that two self-selected groups had been formed? Were those who took the vitamins more generally health conscious and affluent, and might not some other aspects of their life style decrease the risk of spina bifida? Remember that a well-designed scientific study requires that two groups must be created that randomly receive either the vitamin or a placebo.

The ethical problems are obvious. Although they could not be completely certain, many people thought it was very likely that folic acid was the important factor. To be completely certain, there was a need to give placebos to some mothers with a high risk of having a child with a neural tube disorder. If folic acid was the active ingredient, then giving mothers a placebo would result in the birth of children with a serious preventable disorder. In Britain the Medical Research Council decided to fund the study, which took place in seven countries.[19] It was not surprising that some doctors were not prepared to take part because of their ethical concerns.

Each day for the first twelve weeks of pregnancy mothers received a tablet that was either a placebo or contained 4 mg folic acid with or without other vitamins. Those who received the folic acid were 72 per cent less likely to have a child with a neural tube disorder than those who did not. Whereas about 1 per cent of mothers receiving folic acid had a child with a problem, 3.5 per cent of those who did not receive folic acid had an afflicted child. Other vitamins did not influence the likelihood that spina bifida would occur.

As a result of this trial folic acid supplementation starting before pregnancy is now recommended for all women who have previously given birth to a child with one of these disorders. In general, women of child-bearing age should consider the amount of folic acid offered by their diets.

This study provided evidence that the diet of some pregnant women in industrialized countries is poor enough to cause physical damage to the nervous system of their babies. If such major damage can be caused by diet, it is reasonable to consider the possibility that more subtle damage, and hence psychological problems, also reflects poor nutrition.

## *Breast-feeding*

Do breast-fed babies do better than bottle-fed babies? They do in the short term, but not necessarily in the longer term. The origin of the short-term advantage is, however, unclear and its importance uncertain. To study the question you need to measure the rate of development of two groups of infants, one group that has been breast-fed and the other bottle-fed. The data from one of many studies with very similar results will be described.

The most commonly used measure of the stage of development in infants was formulated by an American psychologist, Nancy Bayley. It uses a series of increasingly difficult tasks that can be performed by children of particular ages. The extent to which a child can or cannot perform tasks that can usually be performed by children of their age gives a measure of their rate of development. For example a 3-month-old child will be able to reach for a dangling ring; an 8-month-old will uncover a toy hidden by a cloth; at 9 months cubes will be placed in a cup when requested; a tower of three cubes can be built at 17 months. Although this developmental test was originally designed to estimate intellectual capacity, it is now accepted that it does not predict later IQ scores at all well. Development scales are now used primarily to identify children whose intellectual powers and motor control are not developing normally.

Figure 3.4 shows the mental development of children who had been fed either by bottle or from the breast. The pattern is clear: in terms of mental development, those who have been breast-fed longest develop more quickly in the first two years of life. A similar finding resulted when children were given tests of mental development at ages 3, 4 and 5; performance was better in those who had been breast-fed for longer periods. However, a similar relationship was not found with motor performance. When the school reports of the children were examined at 7 to 9 years, performance was better in maths and English in those who had been breast-fed.

What mechanisms cause breast-feeding to be associated with a developmental advantage? All we have is a correlation, and the

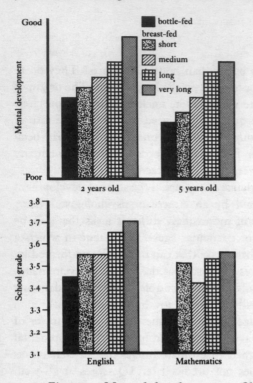

*Figure 3.4* **Mental development of bottle- and breast-fed children**

Children who had been bottle-fed are contrasted with those who had been breast-fed for a short (less than 4 weeks) to a very long (over 20 weeks) period. Development at 2 and 5 years was measured using methods appropriate for the age. School grades for English and mathematics were obtained for children aged 7–9 years: 4 = excellent, 3 = good, 2 = satisfactory, 1 = unsatisfactory.

*Source:* Data from W. J. Rogan and B. C. Gladen, 'Breast-feeding and cognitive development', *Early Human Development*, 31, 1993, 181–93.

problems of interpreting a correlation, discussed in the first chapter, raise their heads. In industrialized countries breast-feeding is more common in mothers who have received longer education and are more affluent. Thus the more rapid development of the breast-fed child may reflect any of a range of advantages. However, attempts to statistically exclude the possibility that the advantage of breast-feeding reflects parental education or social class have suggested that these factors do not explain the phenomenon.

There is always the possibility that the decision to breast-feed is one reflection of a general desire to be a good parent. This would be the case if parents who breast-feed also spend more time with their children throughout their formative years, for example if they were more likely to play educational games and spend more time teaching reading. If this were true, breast-feeding in itself might not have any particular importance.

Apart from offering a source of food, breast-feeding satisfies other needs of the newborn: warmth and security. The baby knows the mother through the smell of the milk and skin. It is easy to look into the mother's eyes and it has been suggested that a strong emotional bond is formed at this time. Bottle-feeding tends to be reported as an emotionally neutral experience whereas breast-feeding is said to be emotionally satisfying for both mother and child. There are reports that breast-feeding mothers talk, touch and smile more while feeding than those using a bottle.[20] There is a general impression that mothers who breast-feed offer the child more stimulation and are more responsive to the child's signals while feeding. It is clear that breast-feeding is a rich interaction that has many dimensions other than the giving of food. It is easy to suggest, and difficult to demonstrate, that this start in life may have consequences for mother–child interaction in later life. The hypothesis that aspects of breast-feeding, other than the composition of the milk, may explain the more rapid development of children has to be taken seriously.

In non-industrialized countries it is widely realized that breast milk can decrease the likelihood of malnourishment in infants born into adverse situations. When 1,000 Tunisian infants born in under-privileged sections of society were examined, those who were breast-fed grew more rapidly in the first twelve months of life.[21] As in industrialized countries, being breast-fed resulted in better performance on measures of development too. The extent to which these differences reflect better nutrition, rather than more general differences in mothering, is unclear. Equally, it must be considered whether in such societies the advantage of breast-feeding reflects, in part at least, a more hygienic method of feeding.

In industrialized societies babies born prematurely are usually fed by a tube that allows milk to be placed directly into the stomach. Such a procedure allows the comparison of the influence of mother's milk and cow's-milk-based formula, as feeding with a tube excludes all the possible benefits associated with a warm, loving mother–child interaction, while allowing any nutritional advantage associated with breast milk. A study directed by Alan Lucas and colleagues at the University of Cambridge followed up a group of premature babies when they reached an age of between $7\frac{1}{2}$ and 8 years.[22] Figure 3.5 shows that the intelligence scores of children who had consumed mother's milk in the early weeks of life were 10.2 points higher. At 18 months the consuming of mother's milk had been associated with more advanced development as judged by the Bayley scale.[23]

The importance of this study is that feeding took place through a tube, removing the possibility that the advantage was due to aspects of breast-feeding unrelated to the milk. The possibility still existed that those mothers who were prepared to express milk for their children had different parental attitudes, or advantages that could have affected the child's development after tube feeding stopped, from those who were happy for artificial feeds to be given. In fact, those who provided breast milk were more likely to come from higher social classes. A way of excluding this possibility is to examine the offspring of those mothers who had wished to breast-feed but were unable to produce enough milk.

It is reasonable to assume that mothers who had wished to breast-feed but had failed had similar attitudes to parenting to those who wished to breast-feed and had been able to produce milk. Was the intelligence of the offspring of the unsuccessful breast-feeders similar to that of those who had managed to breast-feed, in which case differences in parental attitudes would be critical? Alternatively, were the intelligence scores similar to those of the children of parents who had never wished to breast-feed and had received cow's-milk-based formula, in which case the nature of the milk would be important? The answer was that the intelligence of the children of unsuccessful breast-feeders was similar to that of those whose par-

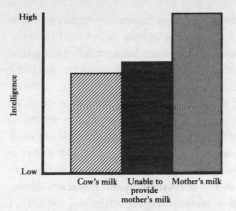

*Figure 3.5* **Intelligence at ages 7–8 of children receiving mother's or cow's milk**
The intelligence of premature babies who received their mother's milk and a cow's-milk-based formula was compared at 7–8 years. The intelligence of children whose mothers had wanted to provide milk but were unable to do so was similar to those whose mothers had wished them to have cow's-milk-based formula, a finding that suggests that parental attitudes are less important than the nature of the diet.

ents had chosen cow's-milk-based formula for their child (Figure 3.5). The most probable explanation was that the higher intelligence at age 8 reflected the consumption of the mother's milk and not parental behaviour. It is, however, very difficult to completely distinguish the effect of breast milk from the fact that mothers from more privileged backgrounds are more likely to breast-feed.

It is unclear what is important in breast milk. Hormones transferred from the mother to the child may play a role, although a nutritional candidate is the provision of long-chain fatty acids that are important in the developing brain. In Adelaide a group in the Flinders Medical Centre evaluated the impact of adding fish oil to infant formula.[24] Fish oils are a source of the essential fatty acids that are needed for brain development. When tested at 30 weeks of age, the visual acuity of those babies who received the fish-oil-enriched infant formula was similar to those who had been breast-fed.

The visual acuity of both these groups of babies was superior to that of babies who had received a traditional cow's-milk-based formula. Although this effect was found in children who were full-term rather than premature, it is unclear whether there are benefits that last beyond 30 weeks of age.

Care should be taken in extrapolating from premature children to those who remain longer inside their mothers. The brains of premature children are less developed. Given that the final weeks of pregnancy are associated with a spurt in the brain's growth, it should not be assumed that breast milk will necessarily prove so influential in those born at the normal time. It is perhaps likely, given the brain's continued development after birth, but it is always possible that certain substances in human milk are important at some stages of the brain's development and not at others. We await further evidence.

## *How can you help your baby's development?*

The strict scientific position is that, excluding gross malnutrition and the fact that taking folic acid supplements decreases the incidence of spinal bifida, you cannot influence the development of your child by your diet. In fact, folic acid may be helpful only in those who have a predisposition to produce children with neural tube problems. Although studies have repeatedly hinted at the possibility that the diet of both the pregnant mother and the newborn infant has developmental implications, few, if any, conclusions may be drawn with any confidence.

In the series of beneficial effects of improved diet that have been described the mothers and children studied were almost always chosen because of their poverty or a history of birth-related problems. It is possible that a similar response would not have been found in better-fed sections of society. When a beneficial response has been found, typically there has been little attempt to relate it to a specific nutritional deficiency. Thus it is impossible to establish the generality of the observations.

The only conclusion that can be drawn is that the situation is complex and poorly understood. It does, however, seem possible that diet will be found to influence development, although its impact may be small and short-lived. Much depends on the stage of the brain's development, what nutrient is of interest and what aspects of motor, mental and emotional development are being considered.

Such a 'fence sitting' conclusion is fine for scientists who have the rest of their lives to consider the topic, and will make a good living out of running further studies. Such a conclusion is, however, unhelpful for parents of a child who is going through a key stage in development. They need immediate advice. It can only provoke anxiety to suggest that diet may indeed influence a child's development but suggest little specific advice.

How can you establish if you are likely to respond to dietary supplementation? If you are short of something in the diet, what is it and how much do you need? There are no means of answering such questions. Conventional wisdom suggests that the vast majority of mothers-to-be who are eating any diet likely to be eaten in an industrialized society do not have a problem.

It is important to keep in perspective the reports that a particular diet in some way speeds a child's development. The positive effects, where they have been reported, tend to be subtle rather than dramatic in nature. The benefits are likely to be short- rather than long-term. Any disadvantage may well be compensated for by other positive experiences of a social or psychological nature. Any nutritional advantage may be lost if other aspects of the environment are not helpful.

After the Second World War an experiment was carried out in Germany that looked at the impact of nutritional supplementation on the growth of children.[25] Identical diets were introduced in two orphanages, Bienenhaus and Vogelsnest. Although the diets were identical, they did not result in an identical weight gain: the children in Bienenhaus grew less. The plan had been to further enrich the diet of the children in Vogelsnest after six months, with the expectation that the rate of growth would increase. Although the children in Vogelsnest had grown more on the original diet, as originally planned they still received the enriched diet, yet they failed to maintain their original advantage. The children in Bienenhaus, who still had the original diet, now began to thrive and their rate of growth increased.

These findings made little nutritional sense. The expectation had been that the children in both orphanages would respond similarly to the basic diet; they did not. The expectation had been that an enriched diet would particularly benefit growth, but the opposite occurred. The answer appeared to be that factors other than nutrition predominated. The home in which the children had failed to thrive had been run by Fräulein Schwartz, who implemented a strict regime. The other home had been run by a loving, motherly matron. By chance, Fräulein Schwartz had transferred from Bienenhaus to Vogelsnest; in both homes, when faced with the harsh regime that she implemented, children failed to thrive, irrespective of the quality of the diet. The exceptions were eight children, who were her favourites, who under both diets had better growth curves than their companions.

Diet needs to be kept in perspective. It may well have a role, but it is not the only factor that influences a child's development. Both physical and mental growth will reflect the social and psychological environment in which the child lives.

Breast milk is nutritionally the most appropriate food for human infants; amongst other benefits, it is a well-balanced food that is easily digested and provides natural immunities. Breastfeeding produces a stimulating and emotionally rewarding interaction that brings short-term benefits. Arguments based on psychological development are less well founded.

Although breast-fed infants develop more rapidly, and in the short term produce higher intelligence scores, the advantages associated with breast-feeding tend to be small and may be of limited long-term significance. If only on the basis that it is just possible that some small long-term psychological benefit will eventually be described, and if not, it will do no harm, breast-feeding can be recommended as the first method of choice. The evidence of long-term psychological benefits is, however, not strong enough for a mother to decide to breast-feed should she feel strongly that she does not want to, or to feel guilty should it prove impossible.

The conservative way forward is to take the common-sense

position that it is just possible that diet may prove important. When pregnant or feeding an infant, particular attention should be paid to what is eaten. It is difficult to offer more specific advice. Clearly most mothers will wish to eat a good diet, but what does this mean? Rather vaguely, it can be suggested that a varied diet should be consumed, one that offers adequate amounts of proteins, essential fatty acids, vitamins and minerals. In the absence of real knowledge, the recommended levels suggested by government bodies are as good an informed guess as any other (see Table 3.2, on p. 50). The general message is that during both pregnancy and lactation there is an increased need for the full range of nutrients.

There is a need to moderately increase the intake of every type of food you eat. If the additional calories all come from one type of food, there is a risk that there may be a short-fall of some nutrients. More specifically, a careful comparison of the British and United States recommendations shows that the figures differ by as much as 75 per cent. If those with access to the scientific literature can only offer rough estimates, it follows that there is no basis for a mother to worry about small deviations from these 'ideals'. Within broad limits, diet should not become an obsession or a cause of anxiety.

*Table 3.2* **Daily recommended dietary requirements[a] of pregnant and lactating women**

|  | Young woman | Pregnant woman | Lactation 1 month | Lactation 6 months |
|---|---|---|---|---|
| Calories (kcal) | 1,940 (2,200) | 2,140 (2,500[b]) | 2,390 (2,700) | 2,410 (2,700) |
| Protein | 45 (46) g | 51 (60) g | 56 (65) g | 53 (62) g |
| **Vitamins** |  |  |  |  |
| Folic acid | 200 (180) μg[c] | 300 (400) μg | 260 (280) μg | 260 (260) μg |
| Niacin | 13 (15) mg | 13 (17) mg | 17 (20) mg | 15 (20) mg |
| Riboflavin | 1.1 (1.3) mg | 1.4 (1.6) mg | 1.6 (1.8) mg | 1.6 (1.7) mg |
| Thiamine | 0.8[d] (1.1) mg | 0.9 (1.5) mg | 1.0 (1.6) mg | 1.0 (1.6) mg |
| Vitamin A | 600 (800) μg | 700 (800) μg | 950 (1,300) μg | 950 (1,200) μg |
| Vitamin $B_6$ | 1.2 (1.6) mg | 1.2 (2.2) mg | 1.2 (2.1) mg | 1.2 (2.1) mg |
| Vitamin $B_{12}$ | 1.5 (2.0) μg | 1.5 (2.2) μg | 2.0 (2.6) μg | 2.0 (2.6) μg |
| Vitamin C | 40 (60) mg | 50 (70) mg | 70 (95) mg | 70 (90) mg |
| **Minerals** |  |  |  |  |
| Calcium | (1,200) mg | (1,200) mg | (1,200) mg | (1,200) mg |
| Iodine | (150) μg | (175) μg | (200) μg | (200) μg |
| Iron | (15) mg | (30) mg | (15) mg | (15) mg |
| Selenium | (55) μg | (65) μg | (75) μg | (75) μg |
| Zinc | (12) mg | (15) mg | (19) mg | (16) mg |

[a] British government recommendations are followed by recommendations of the United States government (in brackets).

[b] Last two-thirds of pregnancy.

[c] μg = microgram, one-thousandth of a milligram.

[d] Last third of pregnancy.

*Sources: Dietary Reference Values for Food Energy and Nutrients for the United Kingdom*, London, HMSO, 1991; *Recommended Dietary Allowances*, Washington, DC, National Academ Press, 1989.

# CHAPTER 4

# Intellectual Growth

It may come as a surprise that after many decades of study psychologists still argue about the nature of intelligence. Initially, some people believed that there was one general dimension of intelligence, although subsequently others have argued that there are several major factors, including verbal, numerical and spatial skills. In the 1920s a statistician, Charles Spearman, found that all tests of mental ability correlated with each other. That is, if you performed well on one test, you tended to do well on other tests. Spearman concluded that these correlations reflected a general factor of intelligence, which he called 'g'. Many years later Raymond Cattell, an Englishman who moved to the United States, argued that there are two types of 'g', which he labelled fluid and crystallized intelligence.

Fluid intelligence is basic problem-solving and reasoning power. It allows deduction and an understanding about the relationship between ideas. Fluid intelligence is viewed as being closely associated with innate, biological potential, and it can be estimated using non-verbal tests.

Crystallized intelligence, in contrast, relies on specific information and vocabulary. It is a reflection of experience and environment. Theoretically, fluid ability provides the native ability that, if it is exposed to learning experiences, allows crystallized intelligence to develop. As people with more fluid intelligence are likely to gain more crystallized intelligence, the two types of intelligence are correlated.

Figure 4.1 gives examples of verbal and non-verbal questions that might be found in intelligence tests. The verbal questions measure crystallized intelligence; vocabulary is clearly a reflection

## Verbal questions

1. Find the word that means nearly the same as the first word in bold type.

**pull**    (a) fix    (b) dig    (c) warm    (d) tug    (e) sell
**jump**    (a) leap    (b) club    (c) refer    (d) rebel    (e) shake

2. Pick the word that best fits the space in the sentence.

Fred likes to ......................... tennis.
(a) talk    (b) play    (c) help    (d) read    (e) call

Water is ................................
(a) dark    (b) green    (c) wide    (d) long    (e) wet

3. Decide how the first pair of words are related to each other and find the missing word that goes together with the third word in a similar way.

hungry – eat   :   thirsty – ......................
(a) beer    (b) wine    (c) drink    (d) bread    (e) glass

big – little   :   large – ...........................
(a) less    (b) grand    (c) great    (d) small    (e) more

4. A series of words are given in bold type. Choose the word that is alike in some way.

**cat   leopard   lion**
(a) panther    (b) dog    (c) horse    (d) bee    (e) donkey

**John   Sid   Frank**
(a) boy    (b) male    (c) Jack    (d) man    (e) Sue

*Figure 4.1* **Verbal and non-verbal questions from intelligence tests**

## Non-verbal questions

1. Find the next in the series.

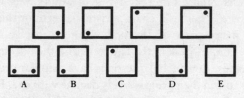

2. Which item completes the grid?

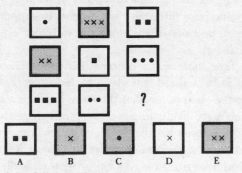

3. Which of the following is similar to:

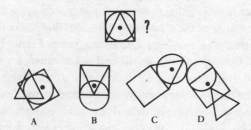

4. Which is the odd one out?

of experience. The non-verbal questions give an index of fluid intelligence. As they do not rely on vocabulary, they tap a basic reasoning ability.

Cattell suggested that one way to demonstrate that verbal and non-verbal tests reflect different types of ability was to monitor changes with age. There is a characteristic pattern for the biological efficiency of many parts of the body. Lung capacity and sexual prowess, for example, peak in the late teens and then decline. Intelligence tests that use non-verbal questions have a similar profile: scores peak at about 20 and then progressively decline with age. In contrast, if you examine performance on verbally based intelligence tests, any decline with age occurs perhaps only forty years after reaching its peak. The profile is so different that it strongly supports Cattell's view that verbal and non-verbal tests tap different aspects of our intellectual make-up.

At one time there was a concern that the intelligence of the population of industrialized societies was declining. The argument was based on the observation that the more intelligent members of the population were likely to have fewer offspring than the less intelligent. The concern was that over generations the gene pool was being diluted and on average we were becoming less intelligent. Even if this had been true, it was not clear what ethically could have been done about it. In fact, it was not true; the opposite was occurring: performance on intelligence tests was increasing rapidly.

Our knowledge of the changing level of intelligence in the population owes a great deal to a New Zealander, James Flynn. He wrote to researchers throughout the world and asked them for any data that they could supply concerning changes in performance on intelligence tests. The findings were very consistent and showed substantial changes. Figure 4.2 illustrates data from three countries. For example, in the Netherlands, for generations, every young man completed the same intelligence test when he started his national service. Thus, with few exceptions, there are test results from the entire male population. Over a period of thirty years intelligence has increased twenty-one points, an enormous change. Flynn was able to find similar evidence from fourteen countries, including the United States, Canada, Japan, Australia, New Zealand, and others in Europe.[1]

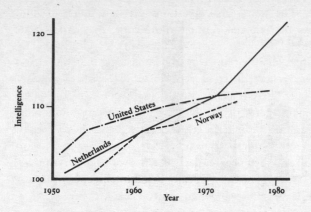

*Figure 4.2* **Increases in intelligence in three countries**
*Source:* Data from Flynn, *Psychological Bulletin*, 101, 1984, 171–91

Clearly, such massive improvements in intelligence test performance must reflect powerful factors, but what are they? Obvious
candidates are better schooling; more verbal stimulation from watching television; greater access to books made possible by increased
affluence. If any of these mechanisms were responsible for the increases, then you would expect that performance on verbally based
tests would be stimulated. Flynn compared performance on verbal
and non-verbal intelligence tests. Figure 4.3 shows such comparisons
in four countries. The results are very clear: it was non-verbal
rather than verbal intelligence that had increased over the decades.
Verbal scores had also increased, but only about half the amount of
the non-verbal scores.

Cattell saw performance on non-verbal intelligence as an index
of biologically based fluid intelligence. Does the very large increase
in non-verbal performance therefore reflect a change in the brain's
basic biology? Richard Lynn, Professor of Psychology at the University of Ulster, thinks that it does; he argues that the increases in
non-verbal intelligence reflect improved diet.[2]

One clue that nutrition may be important is that as intelligence
has increased there have been parallel increases in height. In fact,
the increases in height have been large, about 1.2 centimetres every

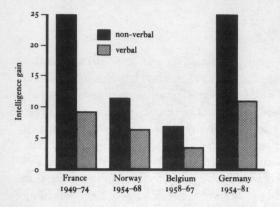

*Figure 4.3* **Relative increases in verbal and non-verbal tests**

Source: Data from Flynn, *Psychological Bulletin*, 101, 1984, 171–91

decade. The most widely accepted explanation for the increase in height is that it reflects improved nutrition, although a reduction in infectious diseases may have played a role, particularly in earlier days.

Richard Lynn considers the hypothesis that the increase in intelligence reflects increased environmental stimulation. When adopted children are examined after moving from biological parents to more stimulating adoptive parents, it is performance on verbal tests that tends to improve. Thus the evidence is that environmental stimulation improves verbal rather than non-verbal scores. Given the evidence that it is non-verbal performance that has dramatically improved over recent decades, this suggests that the underlying mechanism is biological, rather than social, in origin.

The massive increases in intelligence are not experimental observations and it is impossible to establish their origins. At the best all that can be argued is that nutrition is the most likely explanation. In fact, there are interesting parallels between the improvement in performance on non-verbal tests and the response of some children to the provision of vitamin and mineral supplements.

## The Welsh study

In 1987 a short newspaper report of four or five lines stated that Gwilym Roberts, Head of Science at Darland High School, in Wrexham, North Wales, had found that vitamin supplements increased the intelligence of schoolchildren. The reaction of most scientists to such a report would be that such a response was highly unlikely, if not impossible. Nutritional wisdom was that the diet of the vast majority of the population offered sufficient levels of vitamins and minerals. Psychologists would have predicted that an influence, if in fact it occurred, would have been too subtle to have been picked up using a crude, global measure such as intelligence.

I wrote to Gwilym Roberts asking for details of his findings. The details simply confirmed my prejudices. The study had not been double-blind; the study was on too small a scale to produce useful results; there was only the smallest difference in results between those taking the supplement and those taking the placebo. I had offered to subject his findings to statistical analysis, but the difference was so small that there was no point. Gwilym Roberts had, however, been sufficiently encouraged by his preliminary findings to start a larger scale study. He asked if I would help by ensuring that the design and analysis reached accepted scientific standards. Dr Robert Woodward of Larkhall Laboratories had agreed to supply vitamin and mineral supplements and to create placebos. Common sense suggested that I would be wasting my time: there was no research funding and the hypothesis was so extraordinary that it could only lead my academic colleagues to doubt my sanity. I was, however, unaware of any previous study that had examined the psychological impact of giving vitamin supplements to normal schoolchildren. To dismiss the idea without hard data was the act of a bigot. So I became involved, motivated to create a well-designed study that would knock 'such nonsense' on the head. In the event I was to be taught the old scientific lesson that common sense is not always supported by systematic study; that hard experimental evidence should take priority over initial prejudice and theory.

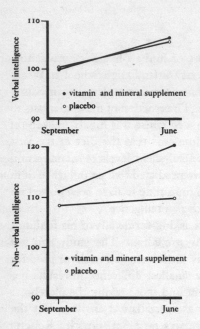

*Figure 4.4* **Impact of vitamin and mineral supplements on the intelligence of Welsh children**
Twelve-year-old children took either a placebo or vitamin and mineral supplement for eight months. Note that non-verbal but not verbal scores increased.
*Source:* Benton and Roberts, *Lancet*, i, 1988; 140–43.

Sixty children took two intelligence tests and then, under a double-blind procedure, received either a placebo or a multivitamin and mineral supplement. After taking the supplement for eight months, they took the tests again. Figure 4.4 illustrates the findings.[3] Performance on the verbal test was not influenced. Scores on the non-verbal intelligence test increased by 9 points after taking the vitamin–mineral supplement, and only by 1.8 points after taking the placebo. The pattern that James Flynn had found in fourteen countries was again found. It was non-verbal rather than verbal scores that had increased.

The response of the academic community on the letters page of the medical journal the *Lancet* was immediate, angry and dismissive. It is very safe to assume that the many letters to the *Lancet* would have pointed out any flaws in the design of the study: they did not. In fact, virtually all comments concerned a dietary survey that did not influence the basic finding that supplementation increased non-verbal intelligence. There were some comments about the statistics that were used, but when the data were subject to independent scrutiny, at the request of the Medical Research Council, these concerns proved to be unfounded. We are left with an unexpected finding that was produced using the widely accepted double-blind approach that is demanded in drug trials.

The data from any scientific study are subject to statistical analysis. The results are expressed in terms of the probability that they might occur by chance. If you spin a coin, there is a 50 per cent chance it will land heads up. If you spin a coin twice, then one time in four you will get two heads in a row. One time in eight you will get three heads in a row, and one time in thirty-two you will get five heads in a row. Traditionally, and arbitrarily, scientists accept their results as valid if they would have occurred by chance less than one time in twenty. When you get unexpected findings there is always the possibility that the result was a statistical freak. Was the improvement in non-verbal intelligence the rogue result that occurs once every twenty times?

In fact, the difference between the Welsh schoolchildren who received the placebo and those who received the supplement was so large that it would have occurred by chance only one time in a thousand. However, given the unexpected nature of the finding, the authors were aware that it might be a statistical freak. Was there something special about the diet of the children they had studied? Would other children respond similarly? Our final comment was cautious: 'Clearly the study must be replicated.' Only if other children were shown to respond would it be reasonable to conclude that there was a genuine response.

## *Attempts to replicate the Welsh findings*

Unknown to the researchers in Wales, a similar study was at the same time in progress in the United States. Steven Schoenthaler is a criminologist who had for many years studied the possible impact of diet on delinquent behaviour. In his latest study he had given twenty-six delinquent juveniles either a placebo or a multivitamin–mineral supplement for thirteen weeks.[4] In this double-blind study no significant change in verbal scores resulted. The non-verbal scores of those receiving the placebo decreased by an average of one point whereas when taking the supplement it increased by six points. The much needed replication had occurred more quickly than expected. The two groups were unaware of each other's findings, or even existence. The similarity of the findings of these two groups created the impression that they were genuine. As Cattell would have predicted, yet again the improvement was on non-verbal and not verbal measures.

In Britain these data received extensive publicity when they were the subject of a television programme entitled 'Your Child's Diet on Trial', broadcast in February 1988 on BBC 1 in the *QED* series. By chance, Tony Edwards, a television producer who specializes in scientific matters, had decided to make a programme on the influence of diet on behaviour. When he began to look around, he learnt of the Welsh and American studies, although only as the programme was being planned did the results become available. The response to the programme was astonishing. The next day most supermarkets and pharmacists in Britain sold out of vitamin supplements. Lorry loads of supplements had to be shipped into Britain from the continent. Several companies launched products with names such as Smart Kid, Tandem IQ and Boost IQ. Throughout Britain parents were giving their children vitamin tablets to increase their intelligence. There is little doubt that the results received too much, and too superficial, media attention.

Scientists entered the race to demonstrate that the phenomenon did not exist: this heresy had to be laid to rest. In King's College London a group that had been very critical of the Welsh research planned a similar study. Under a double-blind procedure children received either a multivitamin–mineral supplement or a placebo for four weeks. 'On retesting there were no significant differences in the performance' and they '. . . found no evidence that learning ability in a cross-section of British schoolchildren was limited by the quality of their diets.'[5]

One reviewer commented that this study only added to the confusion.[6] It was difficult to compare with the original study, it used different tests, different tablets, and took them for a much shorter period. By chance the seven-year-old children who took the placebo were different, in terms of non-verbal intelligence, from those who took the supplement, even before they took the tablets!

A second attempt at replication took place in Dundee at the same time. It tried to faithfully replicate the original Welsh study and reported:

A small, non-significant difference between the control and supplementation groups was found in a non-verbal test. The net difference in changes in scores between the active and placebo groups was 2.4 units. [The] . . . study does not support the hypothesis that vitamin and mineral supplementation leads to improved performance in non-verbal tests of reasoning.[7]

At the same time that these replications were being carried out I was working on a second study, this time in Belgium.[8] Under a double-blind procedure the children were randomly allocated to groups that received either a placebo or a multivitamin–mineral supplement for five months. When verbal and non-verbal scores were examined this time, I initially found no significant differences. What was different? Why had the children in Wrexham and California responded whereas the children in Dundee and London had not?

When studying human behaviour there rarely are simple and universal answers. Typically, not all individuals respond in the same way to the same situation; much depends on their past experience and predispositions. There was an obvious possible explanation. Did the nature of the children's diet determine whether they responded to supplementation? Did those who responded have a poor diet whereas those who did not respond have a better diet?

The children in Belgium recorded everything they ate for fifteen days. The amount of various vitamins offered by the diet was calculated by Professor Buts at the Catholic University of Louvain. Based on these reports, a group of about a third of the boys was selected who consumed significantly lower levels of ten vitamins and minerals. The boys whose diet supplied higher levels of micronutrients did not respond to supplementation. However, the non-verbal intelligence of the boys who ate the poorer diet and received the supplement increased. Again there was no change in verbal intelligence.

Children from seven Belgian schools were studied. The majority, but not all the boys who responded to supplementation, were in the schools for the less academically able children in less economically privileged areas. That the vast majority of the boys who responded were from two of the seven schools illustrates that the choice of subjects is critical. Had the other five schools been studied exclusively, then no response would have been reported. The diets of the Belgian children who responded were significantly worse, in terms of the micronutrients offered, than the diets of the children in both London and Dundee. The workers in Dundee reported that only 6 per cent of their children were as badly nourished as the children who responded in Belgium.[9]

## The DRF study

Graham Aronson was one of the nine million people who watched the television programme. He is a lawyer who specializes in financial matters in Britain and provides financial advice to the government in Israel. With his wife, he controls a charitable trust that specializes in projects that benefit adolescents. The television programme made such a large impact on him that he decided to fund the most extensive and, as it turned out, controversial study on this topic.[10] He established the Dietary Research Foundation (DRF). Not having a scientific background, he set up an international board of advisers. It included Linus Pauling, the Nobel Prize Laureate for chemistry who had in later life advocated orthomolecular psychiatry and that vitamin C will cure the common cold; John Yudkin, Emeritus Professor of Nutrition at King's College London, who had been vociferous in his criticism of the idea that children might respond to micronutrient supplements; Hans Eysenck, Emeritus Professor at the Institute of Psychiatry in London, who has spent his lifetime studying personality and intelligence; and Professor Eric Peritz from the Hebrew University in Jerusalem, who was involved because of his experience of the statistical analysis of large-scale medical studies.

For thirteen weeks Steven Schoenthaler and colleagues ran a trial in which 615 Californian children in their early teens received a placebo or a tablet that contained twenty-three micronutrients at a strength of either 50, 100 or 200 per cent of the United States RDA. The authors of the report concluded: 'Results showed that for non-verbal Wechsler Tests there were highly significant improvements in I.Q., whereas for verbal tests there were none.'[11]

Much of the controversy about the California study resulted from the finding that an improvement in non-verbal intelligence was associated with taking 100 per cent RDA tablets but not with either 50 or 200 per cent of the RDA. This study is the only one that has used more than one dose. It was perplexing that only the 100 per cent RDA tablets produced significant results and for several years this observation caused great doubt to be placed on these findings. It made little sense. If the children responded to 100 per cent of the RDA but not to 50 per cent, you could argue that 50 per cent was not enough. But if they responded to 100 per cent of the RDA, they should also have responded to 200 per cent. Why did they not? Did this imply that 200 per cent was decreasing ability? If too much of the vitamins and minerals had been supplied, the excess would be expected to be simply excreted. If there was no benefit from 200 per cent of the RDA, was there a toxic reaction to these higher doses? In fact, even at 200 per cent of the RDA the dose is low enough for nutritionists to have said that the supplements could be safely consumed.

The answer to these puzzling findings eventually began to become apparent. Both before and after taking the tablets the children had given a sample of blood. These samples had been frozen and, because of the high cost of vitamin analysis, they had been left in the refrigerator. All the money had been used up in collecting the original data. The samples held the answers to the strange pattern of response in the Dietary Research Foundation study, yet the funds to unlock the answers were missing.

Dr Robert Woodward of Larkhall Laboratories came to the rescue. He had supplied the original tablets for the Welsh study and had subsequently sold them under the brand name Tandem IQ. Now he offered to pay for the analysis of the blood samples. The results explained the unexpected pattern of the Dietary Research Foundation findings.[12] In the children who had responded to vitamin and mineral supplements with changes in non-verbal intelligence, there were significantly greater increases in the levels of blood nutrients. Levels can rise only if the body's stores are not already full; that is, if a person is poorly nourished. Those who responded were more likely to have had low blood nutrient concentrations prior to taking the supplements. Importantly, the proportion of children who initially had low levels of vitamins in their body differed between the groups who received 50, 100 and 200 per cent of the RDA. The reason that the children responded to 100 per cent of the RDA was that, by chance, there were more poorly nourished children who were given these tablets. You could use the results of the vitamin analysis to distinguish children in the 50 and 200 per cent RDA groups who were poorly nourished. When this was done, it was apparent that those with low levels of vitamin had responded to supplementation with increased non-verbal scores. Previously, the response of these children in the 50 and 200 per cent RDA groups had been hidden; they were part of a larger group of well-nourished children who had not responded.

A pleasing part of the Dietary Research Foundation study was that some of those involved thought it very unlikely that children's intelligence might respond to supplementation. The presence of sceptical people means that it is likely that the most rigorous of procedures will be followed: they have psychological capital invested in ensuring that the results turn out to be negative. John Yudkin was one of the harshest critics of the Welsh study, although, greatly to his credit, he was open-minded enough to join the Dietary Research Foundation team. In 1988 he commented of the Welsh study:

'This is the most scandalous paper I've seen printed in the *Lancet*. The study is ludicrous meaningless nonsense. They'll take a long time to live this down.'[13]

Following the DRF study that he helped to design, he remarked, 'Our studies show, we believe conclusively, that adding vitamins and minerals to the diets of children who have no obvious physical signs of nutrient deficiency can nevertheless produce an increase in their IQ scores.'[14]

## How adequate are children's diets?

If a response to supplements can be demonstrated, then clearly children's diets cannot be adequate. Is this really so? Dr Roger Whitehead, head of the Dunn Nutrition Unit at Cambridge University, and one of the most influential nutritionists in the United Kingdom, has stated: 'No physiological explanation exists of how vitamin and mineral supplementation could affect brain function in a well-nourished subject.'[15]

It is difficult to question such a tautological statement: if you are well nourished, then, by definition, you will not respond to supplementation. What the comment illustrates is the certainty with which nutritionists assert that people are well fed. The question is whether we can state with total confidence that children are well fed. The problem for nutritionists is that any reliable demonstration that the giving of vitamin–mineral supplements improves functioning leads to the conclusion that they are not well fed. Such a conclusion conflicts with their perceived wisdom.

In Britain many nutritionists will quote the Department of Health survey of the diets of British schoolchildren[16] to demonstrate that there is little or no reason to worry about the nutrition of children. The conclusions that are justified by this study were discussed in Chapter 2, and we have seen that while the average intake of various vitamins reached the accepted standard, there were groups of children who ate less than 70, or even 50, per cent of the RDA (see Table 2.4). All that can be said of such data is that the lower the percentage of the RDA consumed by an individual, the greater the probability that it is inadequate. The acid test to show that somebody is nutritionally deficient is to demonstrate that they respond to supplementation in a double-blind trial.

---

### James: a boy who finds it difficult to concentrate[17]

James was an 8-year-old boy who had been referred to the local educational psychologist because he displayed obsessive behaviour and was unable to sustain attention. The teacher said that he talked a lot and was often out of his seat when he should have been working. His mother commented that he was always eating sweet things and on one occasion had gone to school eating a kilogramme bag of sugar.

The educational psychologist asked a researcher from the local university to help, as he wondered if diet might be a problem. Before taking the supplements, James's IQ was measured as sixty-six; this increased to eighty after taking the vitamins and minerals for six weeks. An increase of fourteen IQ points was greater than had been found by the researchers with any other child in similar studies. Before taking the tablets James spent 39 per cent of his time in the classroom on his school tasks; this increased to 50 per cent after taking the tablets. When faced with a frustrating task, he was more likely to concentrate following supplementation; his parents rated his mood as having improved. Although some of the more objective measures of his behaviour suggested an improvement, his teacher commented that the change was not particularly obvious. The improvements were subtle rather than dramatic. Although the supplementation may have made a small contribution, in no sense had it solved all his problems.

---

In fact, there is no necessary inconsistency between the improvement in non-verbal intelligence in some children and surveys of children's diet. Both suggest that some, but not all, children have a poor diet. There is no suggestion that all children respond to supplementation with improved non-verbal scores. The evidence is that only a minority benefit, those whose diets supply low levels of vitamins and minerals.

Scientifically, the missing link is to measure vitamin status in a group of children and then give vitamin supplements. If the above views are accurate, it should be possible to point to those children who will benefit from supplementation before they start taking the pills. In part, the blood analysis of the DRF study has presented such data, but independent confirmation will add greatly to the confidence that can be placed on the conclusions so far drawn.

Even if you accept the conclusion that some children are badly nourished, many questions remain. What is it that is missing from the diet, a little bit of everything or are particular nutrients important? Are other aspects of psychological functioning disrupted as well as non-verbal intelligence? Is the phenomenon more likely to occur at some stages of development rather than others?

## Blur and slur

Science is far from the systematic and unemotional analysis of experimental data that non-scientists might hope. Even august journals such as the *Lancet* and the *British Medical Journal* published comments on the media attention and sale of supplements initially and only later on the science.[18] Steven Schoenthaler was described as having published his findings 'in an obscure journal'.[19] The news section of *Nature* similarly remarked: 'The journal has a small (less than 1,000) circulation and is edited by Hans Eysenck, a co-author of the study.'[20]

In private, and when commenting anonymously to the press, stronger negative statements have been made. When reviewing a paper for possible publication, a referee for a leading American paediatric journal wrote: 'Was some toxin in the so-called placebo?' The reviewer, unable to point to faults in the design or analysis of the study, makes an accusation of fraud. A similar possibility was openly discussed by a leading British paediatrician at the 1988 Medical Research Council committee that examined the question. Only a few seconds' thought would lead you to dismiss such an accusation. To date, the tablets used in these studies have been produced by five different companies in three different countries, demanding a highly improbable conspiracy. The desire to discount unwelcome findings indeed induces desperate arguments.

## Evaluation

Before attempting to draw conclusions I should declare an interest. I have been responsible for three studies that have found a positive response in at least some children. It should be clearly understood, however, that any suggestion that children respond to vitamin–mineral supplementation with an increase in intelligence scores is far from a statement of scientific orthodoxy. Of ten studies on the topic, seven have reported that taking supplements was associated with improved performance on intelligence tests, or measures of attention, in at least some children.[21] The pattern of changes after supplementation is remarkably constant: when an improvement has been reported, non-verbal rather than verbal measures have increased. Anybody trying to explain away these data has the difficult job of explaining this consistent and selective impact on intellectual functioning.

The theoretical prediction that it would be non-verbal rather than verbal scores that would improve adds to the confidence with which the data may be viewed. On one occasion someone commented that he had taken a vitamin tablet before taking a French examination and it had not made any difference. This is hardly surprising, as it is a totally unreasonable expectation. If taking a vitamin tablet had ever been reported to increase verbal scores, this in itself would be grounds to doubt the finding. The prediction that your vocabulary would increase if you took a vitamin tablet makes little sense.

The implications of the findings are so widespread that it is reasonable to want cast-iron proof. If the phenomemon is accepted, then the way that RDAs are calculated and the levels at present recommended will need to be examined. The issue is political. Which government wants to be told that sections of the population are nutritionally deficient to the extent that their intellectual potential is disrupted? Calls to change economic and social policies would be bound to follow. The food industry has invested heavily in the production of refined, processed foods; the recommendation that you should eat more unrefined, complex carbohydrates is financially unwelcome. Given this list of implications, cautious conclusions are highly desirable.

## What is best for your child?

The scientific approach is to say that something has not been proved until you can be virtually 100 per cent certain of the conclusions. Although we must accept the need for an overwhelming burden of proof when dealing with scientific matters, this is not a practical approach in our day-to-day life. As a parent with a rapidly growing child, I do not have the luxury of the time needed to establish something with certainty. So what should a concerned parent do about vitamin–mineral supplements? Those with growing children may be inclined to accept a lesser burden of proof than a scientist, especially if the implications of doing so lead to changes that will do little harm, if they do little good.

The first thing to do is to look at your children's diet. Nobody suggests that all children will benefit from supplements. If your children have a hearty appetite, will eat anything and you provide a varied, nutritious diet, then in all probability they have no deficiency problems and supplements will have no effect. There is no evidence that vitamin–mineral supplements will improve the intellectual performance of a well-fed child; they will not make anyone supranormal. At the most, they will solve problems caused by a poor diet.

If you have some reason to believe that your children are poorly nourished, should you give vitamin–mineral tablets? In the best of all worlds, definitely not. There is much more to diet than minerals and vitamins. No responsible parent is going to say that I know that my children's diet is inadequate but, as I cannot be bothered to offer appropriate food, I will give pills. To a great extent we eat what we are used to eating. If you establish poor eating habits in childhood, they are likely to continue into adulthood. It would be grossly irresponsible to continue to offer your children a diet that predisposed them to poor health later.

The dietary advice that should ensure that your children do not need to take supplements is essentially the same that is offered to everyone to promote good health: eat more unrefined carbohydrates and fewer of your calories in the form of fat and refined carbohydrates – in particular, sugar; eat at least five to six portions of fruit and vegetables a day. Anybody who has had dealings with children will know that this is easy advice to give and, for many children, difficult advice to take. If you need to change your children's diet, then do it slowly. Introduce a series of small changes rather than a totally new diet all at once. An unfamiliar diet will tend to be rejected. Do not be discouraged if some foods are rejected; try to find others that are acceptable.

How do you know if your child's diet is marginally deficient in vitamins or minerals? Well, you don't. Many children refuse to eat a particular category of foods; vegetables, and meat that does not have a totally uniform texture are two possibilities. Some derive too many of their calories from one source, biscuits or sugary drinks for example. Paediatricians in Southampton described young children who only picked at their food at mealtimes. It turned out that they drank so much fruit squash throughout the day that they obtained the majority of their calories from this source. At mealtimes they had no appetite. Such children are at risk of nutritional deficiency: if too high a proportion of their calories comes from sugar, their intake of micronutrients can be too low. When fruit squash was gradually removed from the diet of the children in Southampton, their appetite returned and the rate of growth increased.

Some children restrict their diets for different reasons. Girls as young as 9 have been found to slim in an attempt to achieve a fashionable figure. There are obviously potential problems for a child going through a growth spurt who limits food intake: if the diet does not supply the basic building blocks, organ damage or stunted or abnormal growth can result. In older children selective diets can be a source of problems. As we saw in Chapter 2, a vegetarian diet has the potential to cause iron deficiency. Any diet that is not varied enough may potentially supply too few vitamins or minerals. Although you can never know if your children are short of micronutrients, a common-sense examination of their eating habits should be able to establish those who are at high risk.

If there is little reason to believe that there is a dietary problem, why not take a supplement as an insurance policy? If you have the money and inclination, then that is your choice. As long as you are aware that it is possible that you are wasting your money, and you do not expect dramatic changes, then in low doses it will do no harm.

There is no reason to expect a dramatic change in your children after they begin taking supplements even if they have a low intake of micronutrients. Remember that we function intellectually using crystallized intelligence, but it was the scores of non-verbal performance that were stimulated by supplementation. Assuming that your children would, in fact, benefit from supplementation, all that you can expect to improve is intellectual potential. Unless that potential interacts with a stimulating environment, it remains as nothing more than potential, something that has not been exploited. Improved nutrition will bring no intellectual gain unless it takes place in a stimulating, emotionally secure environment. Even then the changes will take place gradually over a long period.

# CHAPTER 5

# Food Allergy or Food Intolerance?

Richard Mackarness is a psychiatrist, whose book, *Not All in the Mind*,[1] did much to alert both the public and the medical profession to the possibility that there can be severe adverse reactions to food. His approach was to describe patients whose symptoms had been untreatable for years, but who made a remarkable recovery when common foods were removed from their diet. Mackarness's first controlled case, the study of Joanna, graphically illustrated the serious problems that food can cause.

### *Joanna: nearly a tragedy*

Joanna had first entered a mental hospital following the birth of her third baby and was treated with electro-convulsive therapy. She had become depressed and irritable, was unable to feed the newborn child and rarely changed a nappy. Over a period of seven years she was in and out of psychiatric hospitals thirteen times. On occasions she was violent towards her other two children: she had thrown her daughter through a ground-floor window; she had knocked her $3\frac{1}{2}$-year-old son unconscious. Her tension and depression were sometimes directed towards herself: she would slash her forearms, leaving deep wounds quite unlike the superficial cuts made by those seeking help by making a suicidal gesture.

During this period many of the local psychiatrists had seen Joanna. The difficulty of the case is illustrated by their failure to agree on a diagnosis, and by Joanna's failure to respond to treatment. She had been said to have schizophrenia, schizo-affective psychosis, presenile dementia, temporal lobe epilepsy, neurotic depression and anxiety hysteria. Given that the treatment a person receives depends on the diagnosis that is given, and whether he or she gets better relies on the diagnosis being accurate, it is hardly surprising that the treatments had failed to help with these severe psychotic symptoms.

In May 1973 a case conference was held to discuss Joanna. If she was not continually watched, she was likely to run off and slash herself, often with broken glass. She had failed to respond to a wide range of drugs and various other approaches. In the absence of other alternatives, it was agreed to recommend brain surgery, although the prognosis was not good.

Richard Mackarness, her psychiatrist, had long had an interest in the work on food intolerance and behaviour carried out by several doctors in the United States. Before taking the irreversible step of brain surgery he suggested that the possibility that food was the origin of Joanna's problems be examined. Hippocrates had been aware that food could cause illness. In the 1920s and 1930s American doctors such as Albert Rowe[2] in California, Arthur Coca[3] in New Jersey and Ted Randolph and his colleagues[4] in Chicago had fed restricted diets to subjects to see if their symptoms disappeared. Mackarness and his colleagues used similar methods to examine the possibility that Joanna's behaviour, over many years, had been simply a response to her diet.

Initially, Joanna fasted for five days with nothing but water to drink. The cocktail of heavy doses of six psychiatric drugs was gradually stopped. A record of her usual diet before fasting suggested a high intake of coffee and the possibility of addiction. For the first two days there was a withdrawal period, a hangover during which Joanna felt worse, although by the third day she was much better. She became more co-operative and gave a detailed history that revealed various indications of allergy. For years her nose had itched, her eyes had watered, she had suffered with a rapidly beating heart, she was greatly overweight.

Gradually, different foods were reintroduced into her diet. Steak, green beans and rice produced no reaction, but bacon induced a drop in pulse rate, a wheezy chest and a depression that lasted several hours. When the mood had lifted, Joanna was given eggs, and a really severe response occurred with the risk of self-mutilation. A depressed, downcast posture returned, and Joanna communicated only with difficulty in monosyllables. Food testing proceeded for two weeks, during which it was established that Joanna had a pronounced negative reaction to bacon, egg, porridge, veal, tongue, coffee and chocolate. Her reaction to a food item lasted from six to twenty-four hours.

The next stage was to demonstrate beyond doubt that these were physical, as opposed to psychological, reactions to food. The hospital dietitian blended ten foods with water. Previously, Joanna had been shown to respond to only five of these foods. The foods were administered directly into the stomach using a tube. Only the dietitian had the code saying which food had been administered. Joanna's subjective feelings and the independent impression of two nurses were recorded after a food was given by tube. Only when one food a day had been administered, on each of ten days, was the code revealed. The results were found to be completely consistent with the previous findings: adverse reactions had been observed on the days when the suspect foods were administered, but not on the other days.

The next day Joanna returned to her family without any drugs but carrying a menu that avoided the foods that were unsafe for her to eat. Almost immediately she found a job. Her general practitioner commented, 'Joanna has made a remarkable improvement. She is happy, gay, euphoric . . . she cares for the children without harming them, looks after her house and generally seems to be almost back to her old self . . .'[5]

Joanna's story is a sad one and could so easily have ended in complete tragedy. The emotional impact of such examples helped to convince the public that adverse reactions to food are a problem. The cover of Richard Mackarness's book claimed that it 'shows how millions may be made ill, physically and mentally, by common foods such as milk, eggs, coffee and white flour'.

Can we really draw such a conclusion? Joanna's case, and others like it, clearly demonstrate that food can be one cause of serious psychological problems. Is it, however, reasonable to conclude that food is the basis of the physical and psychological problems of millions in the population? Is Joanna's problem typical of the majority of those in mental hospitals, or is it exceedingly uncommon? Although we use the term food allergy, can we be sure that the problem is allergic in nature? The rest of the chapter is addressed to these and related questions, although no simple answers will be offered.

## What's in a name?

As it is responsible for a great deal of confusion, it is unfortunate that the term food allergy has been so widely misused. In fact, allergy has a narrow and specific meaning that excludes most of the adverse reactions to food: one scientist[6] has distinguished twenty-five separate mechanisms by which food produces such reactions. For our purposes it is simplest to consider these reactions in two categories: food aversion, which reflects psychological mechanisms, and food intolerance, which has biological causes. Table 5.1 suggests a basic distinction between food aversion and food intolerance, and gives some major examples of each.

*Table 5.1* **Causes of adverse reactions to food**

| *Psychological: food aversion* | *Biological: food intolerance* |
| --- | --- |
| Psychological food intolerance | Allergy |
| | Enzyme defects |
| Food avoidance | Fermentation of food residues |
| | Irritants and toxins |
| | Pharmacological reactions |

## Food aversion

### Psychological food intolerance

Psychological intolerance occurs when unpleasant bodily reactions are caused not by the food itself, but by emotional responses that have become associated with the food. A key question is whether the reaction occurs when the food is inadvertently eaten, perhaps in a purée when the appearance and taste are masked or when it is administered directly to the stomach by tube. If there is no response in this situation, but there is a strong reaction when the food item is knowingly consumed, then the reaction must be psychological in origin.

The symptoms are likely to be vague and may vary over time, but, typically, in any individual particular responses will predominate. In addition to feeling generally unwell, specific symptoms may be related to the digestive system, including complaints of swelling or discomfort of the gut, as well as nausea or diarrhoea. Alternatively, palpitations and chest pains may be reported as well as breathlessness or dizziness. When psychological symptoms such as depression, sleep disturbance and irritability occur, they are usually perceived as being secondary to the supposed adverse biological reaction to food.

When people tell their doctor that they respond adversely to food, in many instances the doctor will wonder if the problems are of a minor psychiatric nature and may offer an anxiety-relieving drug. The patient–doctor relationship may well be strained. Subjectively, people will have closely associated the symptoms of anxiety with consuming particular food items. The great deal of media attention given to food-related responses may suggest to them that their own diagnosis is likely to be valid.

Why then is the medical profession so often apparently blind to the seemingly obvious? The examination of relevant experiments answers the question. One such study[7] examined twenty-three patients whose bowel symptoms were suspected of reflecting food intolerance. Objective evidence was sought by using diets that excluded certain food items and then studying the reaction to their reintroduction. In only four out of these twenty-three patients was there a relationship between food and the symptoms. The remaining nineteen were characterized by a high incidence of psychiatric complaints, typically neurotic symptoms and personality disorders.

When faced with patients who claim that they suffer from food-induced disorders, the medical profession must consider two possibilities: that the food causes the problems, and that the belief that food causes the disorder is a reflection of a more general psychiatric problem. There is little question that both these explanations are potentially valid; the difficulty is to establish which is appropriate. The medical profession may be predisposed to dismiss food intolerance because it is statistically unlikely to be the cause of the problem. People, on the whole, are hostile to being described as suffering from psychiatric disorders. In contrast, the suggestion that an external agent such as food explains the problem offers a socially and psychologically acceptable explanation.

### Food avoidance

The second type of psychological response is termed food avoidance. The dividing line between a normal and acceptable degree of food avoidance and an abnormal and unacceptable one – that is, one that has negative nutritional or behavioural consequences – is not clearcut. It will vary greatly from individual to individual because people differ in their needs for particular nutrients.

The general refusal of a young child to eat may be the reflection of a general negative attitude to life and can easily become a battle of wills. A child may be seeking more autonomy whereas the parent is concerned about adequate nutrition. Parents, with the advantage of emotional maturity, should not associate the refusal of food with rejection of parental love.

There can be few, if any, children who do not at some stage express food likes and dislikes. The forms are many and varied, but may consist of a refusal to eat all of one class of food, such as vegetables, or an insistence on eating only a limited range of foods, such as chips, biscuits or soft drinks. If food fads are extreme and prolonged, the danger arises that a balanced diet is not consumed.

Reserves of vitamins and minerals may be exhausted. If this scenario is likely to occur, then the use of vitamin–mineral supplements should be considered, although it should be remembered that the bodily reserves of some of these nutrients last for months.

Social and cultural pressures are largely responsible for widespread dieting amongst both the adolescent and adult population. There is a conflict between the fashion-dictated lean and angular female shape and affluence that offers plentiful calories. For the teenage girl in particular, adolescence is a time of growth, fashion consciousness, preoccupation with body shape and weight, and emotional immaturity. If carried to extremes, dieting may predispose a person to potentially life-threatening eating disorders, such as *anorexia nervosa*, which is characterized by a pathological fear of food.

Dieting inevitably involves avoiding particular types of food, typically those containing carbohydrate and fat. Even when carried out in a very moderate manner dieting can result in an unbalanced diet. For example, breakfast cereals are commonly avoided for their carbohydrate content, but in many diets this is an important occasion when milk is consumed. As milk is an important source of calcium, a seemingly minor food avoidance can have important nutritional consequences. A long-term low calcium intake can lead to demineralization of bone, with an increased risk of broken bones in older women.

## Food intolerance

The generic term 'food intolerance' is used to imply that although there is an adverse reaction to a food, there are many possible mechanisms. Figure 5.1 summarizes the wide range of possible symptoms. The majority of symptoms associated with food intolerance are physical, although some, for example depression, anxiety and hyperactivity, are psychological in nature. Although it is beyond the scope of this book to discuss the possible physical symptoms associated with food intolerance, it should be noted that the topic generates a great deal of controversy.

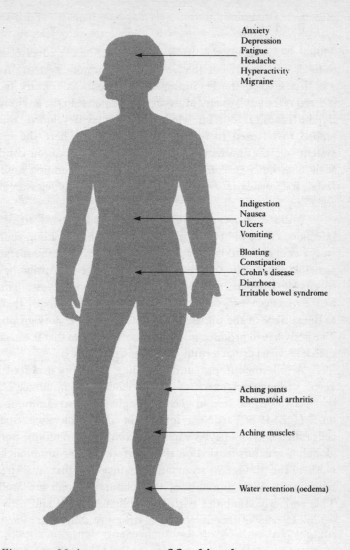

Anxiety
Depression
Fatigue
Headache
Hyperactivity
Migraine

Indigestion
Nausea
Ulcers
Vomiting

Bloating
Constipation
Crohn's disease
Diarrhoea
Irritable bowel syndrome

Aching joints
Rheumatoid arthritis

Aching muscles

Water retention (oedema)

*Figure 5.1* **Main symptoms of food intolerance**

### Food allergy

Although 'food allergy' is often used to describe any adverse reaction to food, it is strictly one that involves the immune system. 'Allergy' was first used at the beginning of the twentieth century to mean 'altered reactivity', or any idiosyncratic response to the environment. By the 1920s, as our knowledge of allergies developed, the term tended to be used to include only reactions where the immune system was the mechanism of action. In this tradition conditions such as asthma, eczema, non-seasonal rhinitis (running nose), hay fever and urticaria (nettle-rash) are known as classic allergic reactions.

Antibodies are proteins produced in the body to fight off infections. They bind to a virus and stop it from invading your cells. In the case of bacteria they need help, so they coat the surface and signal to other cells that are able to kill bacteria. Antibodies bind specifically to a particular target cell. If, for example, you are infected by the measles virus, your body makes a specific antibody that binds to the surface of the measle virus but not to other foreign proteins. The body has to produce millions of antibodies so that it can combat each new virus or bacterium that enters the body.

A milestone in our understanding of allergy occurred in the 1960s with the discovery of the antibodies, or immunoglobulins, that play a central role in classic allergic reactions. Immunoglobulin E (IgE) is of particular interest in food intolerance. Specialist cells called B-lymphocytes each produce their own unique immunoglobulin, which is carried on their surface. If that immunoglobulin binds to the protein on an invading pathogen – that is, a virus or a bacterium – large amounts of the immunoglobulin are produced. This antibody combines with the foreign proteins and activates a complex series of reactions that destroy invading micro-organisms (Figure 5.2).

While attacking foreign substances, the host body also suffers. For example, IgE, after being produced by the B-lymphocytes, binds to the surface of mast cells. Mast cells are found throughout the body but are particularly common in the tubes leading to the lungs, the nose and the gut. They are positioned to defend the body

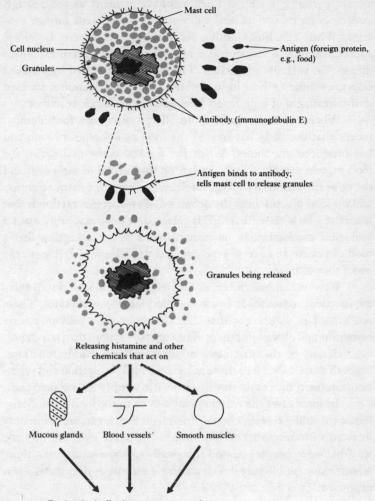

*Figure 5.2* **An allergic reaction**

A food protein (an antigen) binds to an antibody on the surface of a mast cell. Histamine and other chemicals are released that cause allergic symptoms.

against parasites. Each mast cell will have as many as 100,000 IgE molecules on its surface and will respond to different foreign proteins. When IgE binds with a foreign protein, mast cells release substances such as histamine, serotonin and prostaglandins, which inflame the surrounding tissues. The chemicals released by the mast cells are similar to those in insect bites, and anti-histamines are used in the treatment of both insect bites and some allergic reactions.

When the body reacts in an allergic way to a food item, it means that the body has treated the food as a foreign protein and has produced antibodies. When the food is consumed again, the food protein combines with the IgE on the surface of mast cells and the powerful chemical cocktail is released. Today, for many scientists and medical practitioners the definition of an allergic reaction is that laboratory tests show that IgE is released. They reasonably want a biological mechanism to be demonstrated before accepting that a food can cause an adverse reaction, and the release of IgE gives the proof they require.

However, although IgE is involved in most food-induced allergic reactions, some foods cause so-called false food allergies. These foods contain substances that directly cause mast cells to release histamine and other substances. The cocktail of more than ten chemicals released by the mast cells influences various bodily functions. Smooth muscles, such as those associated with respiration and digestion, contract; the result may be asthmatic symptoms and diarrhoea.

In some cases the reaction may not be to the food itself. Many foods, including cereals, cheese, dried fruit and sugar, are commonly infested with mites that are invisible to the naked eye.[8] In the same way that many people respond allergically to house-dust mites, those who are susceptible may develop allergic asthma or dermatitis when exposed to food mites.

## Pharmacological reactions

Caffeine, which is found naturally in tea, coffee and cocoa, and is an ingredient in some cola drinks, is the most widely used stimulant in the world and as such is the most obvious pharmacologically active agent we consume. Caffeine is addictive and has widespead effects on the body, including stimulation of both the brain and heart (see Chapter 12). It also stimulates urine output and dilates the lungs. Consuming large doses of caffeine can produce nausea and even vomiting in susceptible individuals. Given its profile of action, it is not surprising that, if taken in too large quantities, caffeine induces symptoms similar to an anxiety state: tremor, sweating, rapid breathing, palpitations.

In many foods there are chemicals that, similarly to caffeine, act on blood vessels and either directly or indirectly release adrenaline and a related chemical, noradrenaline, from nerve endings. Such foods include cheese, yeast extracts, wine and bananas. The active chemicals include tyramine, serotonin and histamine. Histamine is stored in granules in mast cells, from which it is released in allergic reactions. It also is a normal constituent of fermented foods, such as cheese, although the amounts present are usually small unless bacterial action has continued in old samples. There are, however, reports of intoxication following the eating of cheese containing high concentrations of histamine.[9] The symptoms of histamine intoxication include nausea, vomiting, headache, difficulty in swallowing, thirst and an itchy nettle-rash-like reaction (urticaria).

Dry fermented sausages, such as pepperoni and dry salami, tend to have higher levels of histamine than sausages that have been cooked, although the nature of manufacture and storage is important. Fish of the mackerel family if badly stored may contain high levels of histamine that are responsible for a response that is indistinguishable from an allergic reaction (scombrotoxin illness). The storage of mackerel at o °C ensures that histamine levels remain low; at room temperature the amounts present can rapidly rise to toxic levels, although the fish may appear edible.

Fermented cheese, such as blue Stilton, and a number of other foods also contain high levels of tyramine, which can cause the release of noradrenaline, which, in turn, increases blood pressure. Normally, the liver rapidly breaks down tyramine and the changes in blood pressure are unimportant. However, serious problems can arise in people taking one of a group of anti-depressant drugs known as monoamine oxidase inhibitors (by no means the most commonly prescribed anti-depressants). In the presence of these drugs the tyramine present when large amounts of cheese, chocolate, liver, sausage or yeast extract are eaten increases blood pressure to the extent that headaches, dizziness and severe nausea may result; a cerebral haemorrhage or heart failure can occur.[10]

About half of all people with a food intolerance crave the foods that cause their symptoms, although if the craving is for common foods, such as milk or wheat, this may go unnoticed. A possibility that has recently emerged is that some foods may act in a similar way to opiate drugs. The gut and the brain contain small proteins (peptides) that are known as endorphins (contraction of 'endogenous morphines'), which act at the same sites as morphine and heroin. The incomplete digestion of food proteins can result in the production of chemicals called exorphins, which mimic the action of endorphins. Why might some people respond to food in this way and others not? Nobody knows, but there is some evidence that the permeability of the gut is greater in some individuals, allowing more peptide into the bloodstream. Alternatively, there may be individual differences in the amount of the enzymes available to break down the exorphins. Partially digested milk, wheat and maize have been shown to contain these exorphins. Although conclusive proof that exorphins produce addictive eating is not available, it remains an interesting idea.

## Enzyme deficiencies

The sugars sucrose, maltose and lactose are broken down by the enzymes sucrase, maltase and lactase in the small intestine. Without these enzymes, sugars are not broken down and will enter the large intestine, where they attract water, causing diarrhoea. They may also ferment, and the resulting gas will cause discomfort.

Only humans drink milk after weaning and as such are the only species to consume the milk sugar, lactose. As they have no need to break down lactose, most adult mammals have the enzyme lactase to only a very limited extent. The majority of adult humans, like other mammals, have very little lactase and therefore avoid raw milk; in many parts of the world milk is consumed in the form of yoghurt, after the lactose has been broken down by bacteria. The

## *Joyce*

Joyce was 63 and had suffered from depression for many years; at one stage the problem was so bad that she had been admitted to a mental hospital. She complained of abdominal pain, was bloated and suffered with diarrhoea. Her doctor diagnosed irritable bowel syndrome and told her there was nothing that he could do. On the recommendation of a friend, Joyce went to another doctor, who put her on an elimination diet. After about two weeks her bowel functioning returned to normal for the first time in several years. When she returned to her normal diet, a clear pattern was observed. If she ate cereal with milk for breakfast, as she had throughout her life, she was bloated by lunchtime, had a bout of diarrhoea in the afternoon and felt profoundly depressed for the next two days. Excluding milk from her diet allowed Joyce to live free from both physical and psychological symptoms.

---

exceptions are most people of European origin, and the very few people in Africa and Asia of Hamitic ancestry.[11] In Britain just under 5 per cent of people of European stock lack the enzyme to break down the sugar in milk.[12] The ability of most Europeans to consume large amounts of milk as adults shows the importance that the domestication of cattle played in their evolution. Those able to consume milk were more likely to survive and pass on their genes to the next generation.

A lactase deficiency does not, however, mean that modest amounts of milk will not be tolerated. At four months a kitten will stop producing the enzyme but as an old cat still likes a small amount of milk. Hindu culture traditionally emphasizes the role of milk in a good diet, yet only a negligible amount of lactase is present in the intestine of Indians. If milk is drunk in large amounts, a reaction will occur, but not if it is consumed in small quantities. In fact, in Europe an adverse reaction to milk, when it occurs, often does not reflect the absence of lactase.

Very rarely, people lack the enzyme sucrase and are unable

to break down sucrose. Infants with the disorder have chronic diarrhoea and fail to develop until sucrose is excluded from the diet. The role of sucrose intolerance in the hyperactivity in children is considered in Chapter 7.

## Which foods cause reactions?

A great many foods have been reported to be the cause of food intolerance. Table 5.2 lists the more common food items as well as those that are less frequently a source of trouble. Fortunately, the adverse reaction to food is idiosyncratic, so few people, if any, need to avoid everything on the list.

It is useful to distinguish symptoms of an allergic nature, such as asthma, eczema, swelling and rashes, from those associated with the bowel. Evidence of a true allergic reaction, that is the production of IgE antibodies, occurs in about three-quarters of people who react to eggs, fish and nuts.[13] In contrast wheat, corn, dairy products, coffee, tea and citrus fruits are typically associated with bowel symptoms. Milk, dairy products, wheat and chocolate are potentially capable of causing both allergic reactions and bowel symptoms.[14]

Although many adverse reactions to food result in physical symptoms, there have been suggestions that psychiatric symptoms, particularly irritability and depression, may be associated with food intolerance. However, it would be surprising if a psychological reaction to physical symptoms did not occur. People who are in pain tend to be irritable and those who are ill for a long time are predisposed towards depression. The physical mechanisms of allergic reactions can lead to psychological problems; for example, a shortage of oxygen following an asthma attack may disrupt the brain's functioning. Although the report of the Royal College of Physicians concluded that it remains to be demonstrated that food intolerance provokes psychiatric symptoms directly,[15] it is difficult to believe that the authors had considered cases such as Joanna's. There is little doubt that, one way or another, food can dramatically influence behaviour in some people.

*Table 5.2* **Foods that cause food allergy and intolerance**

---

*Foods commonly involved*

---

Artificial colours
Cereals (corn, oats, wheat, rye)
Chocolate
Coffee and tea
Cow's milk
Fish and shellfish
Hen's egg
Pork/bacon
Preservatives
Tenderized meat
Yeast

---

*Other foods reported to cause reactions*

---

| | | |
|---|---|---|
| Aniseed | Clove | Nutmeg |
| Apple | Fennel | Peach |
| Artichoke | Filbert | Peas |
| Banana | Garlic | Peppers |
| Beans (various) | Ginger | Potato |
| Beetroot | Herbs (bay, | Seeds (caraway, |
| Berries (various) | sage, thyme) | dill, poppy, |
| Celery | Honey | sunflower) |
| Camomile | Hops | Sesame |
| Chestnut | Horseradish | Soya |
| Chicken | Mango | Sweet potato |
| Chicory | Millet | Tapioca |
| Cinnamon | Mustard | Vanilla |

---

## How common is food intolerance?

The only way to reliably assess how commonly food intolerance occurs would be to take a representative sample of those who are ill, subject them to an elimination diet, and if the symptoms improve, systematically reintroduce food items. It is hardly surprising that this type of study has not been carried out. Instead, we can only guess at the magnitude of the problem; we are left with the impressions of individuals. Mackarness estimated that 30 per cent of the problems seen by general practitioners are exclusively due to food and chemical allergy.[16] In addition he believes that these mechanisms are in part to blame in another 30 per cent, leaving the remaining 40 per cent whose symptoms are completely unrelated to food. Although similar estimates are echoed by other doctors who believe that food is a common problem, there is little evidence to support this impression.

When systematically studied, estimates of adverse food reaction have repeatedly been found to be too high. The experience of consultants who specialize in adverse food reactions is that a significant proportion of those who believe that they respond adversely to food are displaying a psychological rather than a biological response. David Pearson of Manchester University studied twenty-seven patients who had irritable bowel syndrome and believed it was caused by food intolerance. When the impact of various foods was examined systematically, only 15 per cent were found to respond to food. When these patients were studied by a psychiatrist, 85 per cent had problems of anxiety and depression. The conclusion drawn was that the bowel problems reflected psychiatric rather than food-induced problems.[17] Impressions of the impact of diet can be misleading; there is no substitute for systematic study.

The training of doctors leads many of them to discount the possibility that medical symptoms reflect food-related problems. The characteristics of food intolerance are not those that the medical profession expect of a medical disorder. In the early nineteenth century doctors used the theory of 'miasmas' to explain the patterns of disease. Miasmas were vaguely defined atmospheric conditions, for example cold air, that by uncertain means caused disease. The impact of these atmospheric conditions was non-specific, as some people suffered with cholera, some with typhoid and some with other disorders. Later in the nineteenth century the development of the germ theory by Robert Koch in Germany and Louis Pasteur in France revolutionized medicine. It became apparent that a specific bacterium caused a specific illness. From that time each disease had a specific cause and was characterized by a specific set of symptoms.

In the area of food intolerance no two people are alike. Different foods are a problem for different individuals; the range of symptoms affect most areas of the body; there is not even one symptom that is common to all patients; there are no unequivocal tests for food intolerance; there is no obvious mechanism; people appear to respond to things other than food, such as house-dust mite, pollen and perfumes.

The symptoms are so often of such a general nature that they can potentially reflect a wide range of other causes. That the symptoms are often those associated with psychosomatic and minor psychiatric illness causes additional doubts. It is understandable that there is a reluctance to accept the idea that food acts in such a non-specific and unpredictable way. For many medical professionals the concept of food intolerance, at least given our present level of understanding, is a step backwards to discredited woolly forms of thinking. The history of medicine is of a long series of now discredited cures that were believed to help a wide range of unrelated disorders. In the nineteenth century hydrotherapy required the drinking of large volumes of water and the taking of hot and cold baths. The result was a 'strengthening of the fibres' and the 'removal of poisons'. The giving of mild electric shocks was recommended for nervous afflictions. It is easy to see parallels between such treatments and food intolerance. Some doctors exclude the idea of food intolerance because invoking diet as the cause of a medical problem is intellectually alien to them, the province of cranks and charlatans.

Within traditional medicine the estimate of the incidence of food intolerance is several orders of magnitude lower than that found in popular books. It is estimated that between 0.5 and 1 per cent of the population of the European Union display food intolerance, of whom only some will have a true food allergy. These figures are still a matter for concern: a problem afflicting one in a hundred deserves to be taken seriously. Although such estimates reflect the number of individuals treated for various complaints by the medical profession, they still have the status of an informed guess. We simply do not know how many people are, like Joanna and Joyce, because of misdiagnosis totally unaware that food is the basis of their problem.

However, while it is extremely unlikely that Joanna and Joyce are unique, they are probably not typical cases either. For the individual the frequency with which the problem occurs in the general population does not matter; you either have the problem or you do not. Your concern is that, when appropriate, the possibility of food intolerance is explored.

## So you think you suffer from food intolerance

Having read this chapter you may be thinking that you or a member of your family responds adversely to some foods. What should you do about it? First, think again. The probability is that you do not, but instead are displaying 'Medical Students' Complaint'. Some medical students have the tendency to believe that they have the symptoms of whatever they have been told about in the latest lecture. On the other hand, if you still suspect that you do respond adversely to something in your diet, and particularly if you have severe symptoms that have been resistant to conventional medical treatment, then the possibility is worth exploring.

The methods used are so simple that there is no technical reason why you could not make a preliminary examination by yourself; in fact, several popular books suggest that you do just this. They recommend that you eat a restricted diet and see if the symptoms disappear, then systematically reintroduce food items while you monitor the symptoms. There are, however, several reasons why you would be well advised to seek medical advice first. Firstly, the symptoms that you display will probably be consistent with other disorders: it is sensible that a range of medical checks are made to exclude any more obvious explanations. Secondly, in sensitive individuals the reintroduction of a food item can result, rarely, in anaphylactic shock. This is a severe and rapid allergic reaction in which an antigen–antibody reaction releases large quantities of histamine. The resulting widespread dilation of blood vessels causes a severe fall in blood pressure, which fortunately responds well to the administration of adrenaline. Although anaphylactic shock is rare, it can be fatal. If you have ever had a severe reaction to food in the past, then you should be aware that another exposure may produce an even more serious reaction. In particular, if a food has ever produced a difficulty in breathing, swelling of the lips and tongue or a generalized rash, you would do well to avoid that food completely.

A third reason to seek advice is to ensure that any new diet is not, in turn, the source of problems. The simple solution to an adverse reaction to a food item is to remove it from the diet. However, if for example you remove milk and milk products from your diet, you must ensure that you consume an alternative source of riboflavin and calcium. There have been cases where self diagnosis and the eating of a restricted diet have resulted in severe malnutrition. The advice of a dietitian is invaluable in this context and for help in constructing a diet free from particular food substances. You can be referred to a dietitian by a general practitioner or hospital doctor.

Trying to convince the doctor that your symptoms may be food related may put you in a Catch-22 situation. If you go complaining of neurotic symptoms, how can you convince the doctor that the problem is food related? A good start may be to keep a diary of what you eat and the severity of particular symptoms on various days, perhaps rated on a ten-point scale. Remember that symptoms may appear only after several hours. Such a diary will not prove that you have a problem, but it may help you get the possibility treated seriously; it also suggests that your request is well considered and not merely a hysterical outburst.

## *What can we conclude?*

Adverse reactions to food are generally accepted phenomena. Equally, there is little doubt that when they do occur, they can result in serious problems, of both a physical and psychological nature. There is also general agreement that the reaction may result in varied symptoms afflicting the skin, nervous system, digestive system, cardiovascular system, endocrine glands, muscles and joints. However, it is apparent that the symptoms of food-related complaints overlap with much of the rest of medicine, with many disorders that are unrelated to diet. It is therefore difficult to distinguish food-related complaints from those with other origins. A key question, and one to which there is no clear answer, is how frequently do these adverse reactions to food occur? Traditional medical opinion is that they are relatively rare; others believe that they are very common.

# CHAPTER 6

# Hyperactivity: a Reaction to Additives?

... But Fidgety Phil,
He won't sit still,
He wiggles and giggles,
And then, I declare,
Swings backwards and forwards,
And tilts up his chair,
Just as a rocking-horse –
'Philip! I am getting cross!'
See the naughty, restless child,
Growing still more rude and wild,
Till his chair falls over quite,
Philip screams with all his might . . .[1]

This poem by Heinrich Hoffman, a German physician, is part of the first recorded description of a hyperactive child, one who typically is overactive, impulsive, excitable and easily distracted. Hyperactivity manifests itself at an early age, and aggressive, antisocial behaviour and specific learning problems often develop. There can be few parents who have not on occasion wondered if their child has at least some of the symptoms of hyperactivity, even in a mild form. When hyperactivity is mentioned, it is rarely long before somebody suggests that the child is responding to food colourings or other additives. Is this reasonable? What is the evidence that additives are the cause of this childhood problem?

When trying to determine if a child is hyperactive, a professional will have carefully described diagnostic criteria and the experience of previous assessments. The Conners rating scale (Table 6.1)

*Table 6.1* **Conners rating scale for hyperactive behaviour**

|  | Not at all | Just a little | Pretty much | Very much |
|---|---|---|---|---|
| Restless or overactive | | | | |
| Excitable, impulsive | | | | |
| Disturbs other children | | | | |
| Fails to finish things | | | | |
| Short attention span | | | | |
| Constantly fidgeting | | | | |
| Inattentive, easily distracted | | | | |
| Demands must be met immediately | | | | |
| Easily frustrated | | | | |
| Cries often and easily | | | | |
| Mood changes quickly and drastically | | | | |
| Temper outburst | | | | |
| Explosive and unpredictable behaviour | | | | |
| Scoring | 0 | 1 | 2 | 3 |

Tick the column that most appropriately describes the behaviour of the child and add up the scores. Any child scoring more than 15 is likely to be diagnosed as hyperactive.

*Source:* C. K. Conners, *Feeding the Brain*, Plenum Publishing Corp., 1989, p. 241.

is frequently used in hyperactivity research, and may help to distinguish the naughtiness of normal children from more serious behavioural problems.

All hyperactive children do not display the same symptoms; in fact, there is not one symptom that is central or universally present. The list of possible symptoms is long and clearly represents a problem for both child and parent. The child may be hyperactive, never quiet but running and dancing around, legs and arms rarely stationary. The child may be impulsive or aggresssive and when demands are not instantly met, she or he will react with a tantrum or tears. There may be an inability to concentrate, so the child never sits still throughout a meal, TV programme or task at school. Poor co-ordination may result in clumsiness to the extent that it makes buttoning clothes and writing difficult. Sleep may be a problem; the child is difficult to get into bed, slow to fall asleep and awakens easily. It is hardly surprising that these symptoms are associated with school failure, although typically the child's IQ is normal or above average.

## Why use additives?

Once a diagnosis of hyperactivity is made, parents will want to know the cause and if there is a cure. A survey in the United Kingdom found that over half the population checked food labels to avoid foods with long lists of additives.[2] A visit to any supermarket will demonstrate the response to this concern: labels are prominently displayed that proclaim 'No artificial colours' or 'Contains only natural ingredients'. Leading supermarket chains have widely publicized that they have removed additives from their own branded goods. Some local authorities, for example Birmingham, have banned selected additives from school meals. The reaction of the food industry is largely a reflection of market forces – it finds that the removal of additives is a powerful selling point – and partly the result of direct lobbying by pressure groups concerned, in particular, about hyperactive children.

In 1984 the European Community (EC) required that additives be listed on packaged foods. Figure 6.1 shows the type of lists that resulted, particularly on highly processed convenience foods. For the first time attention was drawn to the chemicals that were being added to food. These were not new additives, but newly declared additives.

> *Ingredients:* Sugar, wheatflour, animal and vegetable fats, whole egg, glucose syrup, chocolate flavour coating (sugar, vegetable fat, whey powder, fat reduced cocoa powder, wheatflour, emulsifier E322, flavouring), skimmed milk powder, rice flour, salt; colours E102, E122, chocolate brown HT, E142; egg white, flavouring, preservative E202; emulsifiers E471, E477; modified starch.
>
> Label of fondant fancies, 1986
>
> *Ingredients:* Modified starch, dried glucose syrup, salt; flavour enhancers monosodium glutamate, sodium 5-ribonucleotide; dextrose, vegetable fat, tomato powder, hydrolysed vegetable protein, yeast extract, dried oxtail, onion powder, spices, flavouring; colours E150, E124, E102; caseinate, acidity regulator E460; emulsifiers E471, E472(b); antioxidant E320.
>
> Label of oxtail soup, 1986
>
> *Ingredients:* Sugar, modified starch, starch, skimmed milk powder, hydrogenated vegetable oil, whey powder, caseinates, salt, emulsifier E471; colours E102, E110, E127; flavourings.
>
> Label of custard mix, 1986

*Figure 6.1* **Ingredients of highly processed foods**
The ingredients are listed in the order of the amount included, with
that in the largest quantity listed first.
*Source:* G. Cannon, *The Politics of Food*, London, Century, 1987, p. 61.

The food we eat has been transformed, particularly since the 1950s. At the beginning of this century only about fifty additives were used, mainly to colour food, mask the use of poor quality ingredients or increase shelf life. Today about 3,800 additives are being used for a multitude of purposes: as bleaches, solvents, foam-reducing agents, preservatives, antioxidants, emulsifiers as well as colours and flavours.[3] The aim is to make products that are cheap, look attractive, have a nice texture, taste and smell good to eat, can be mechanically processed and packaged, and can be displayed on the shelf for long periods without putrefying or changing appearance.

The European Common Market introduced the E-number

system to provide a convenient shorthand way of identifying additives without filling food labels with long chemical names. The unintended consequence was an increased public awareness of the ways in which the food industry had used the skills of the chemist to fill the supermarket shelves. There are 149 additives with the prefix E classified according to use:

E100–180: colours
E200–297: preservatives
E300–321: antioxidants
E322–495: emulsifiers, stabilizers, thickeners.

In addition, 500 to 578, without E numbers, refer to processing aids that help during manufacture, for example by preventing powders from forming lumps or food sticking to the machinery. Numbers 620 to 637 are flavour enhancers, of which 621, monosodium glutamate, is a frequently used example. Finally, bleaches are numbered 920 to 927 and are used, for example, to produce even whiter flour. The list of additives does not stop here, as there are about 3,500 unnumbered flavours as well as enzymes, solvents, modified starches and sweeteners. In many cases the food label does not fully list the additives; a term such as 'added flavours' may cover dozens of chemicals.

The public reacted strongly when the media and popular books stressed the possible adverse reaction to such substances. It was alleged that additives influence a wide range of physical problems, including asthma, rashes, migraine, cancer, and kidney and liver damage. In some cases the scientific evidence was strong enough to lead to the banning of particular additives; in most cases the evidence was weak. Although such physical problems are naturally a cause of concern, they are beyond the scope of this book. However, one of the characteristics most linked with additives still permitted in food is behavioural: hyperactivity in children.

Part of the response of the food industry to public concern has been to change from artificial to natural additives, with the unstated implication that natural additives are unquestionably safe. The word 'natural' has been hijacked by the food industry and used in a way that amounts to a confidence trick. A chemical is a chemical; it matters not at all if it was produced by a plant or in a chemist's test tube. The same question arises in both instances: is it safe to include it in food? Although a natural additive must be found in a plant, it need not be anything that has ever been eaten. Why should it be considered natural to eat a high concentration of one chemical from a never-before-eaten seed of an obscure tree? These alternative additives are as likely, or unlikely, as synthetic additives to be the cause of problems. The idea that everything natural is wholesome and good for you is obvious nonsense: some of the most potent poisons known are derived from plants. In all cases, both natural and synthetic chemicals must be monitored for their possible adverse actions.

## Fleas, food and Feingold

When the influence of additives on children's behaviour is discussed, the Feingold diet tends to be mentioned. Dr Benjamin F. Feingold had practised as both a paediatrician and an allergy specialist for more than twenty years when, in 1951, he became chief of the Department of Allergy in the Kaiser-Permanente Medical Care Program in San Francisco. The new job gave him an opportunity to satisfy his ambition to do some research. For many years this was more to do with fleas than food, and illustrates the serendipitous nature of research: often the more important discoveries are made while studying apparently unrelated topics. Whether Feingold made an important discovery is, however, a continuing controversy.

Many people living in the Golden Gate area of San Francisco requested both treatment for, and protection from, the flea-bite reaction to a particularly virulent local insect. Eventually, it was shown that the reaction to the bite was induced by a chemical in the insect's saliva. In immunology a chemical with a low molecular weight is known as a hapten; it was such a molecule that was injected by the flea. Because of its small size, a hapten is unable to stimulate an immune or allergic response. However, when a hapten combines with a protein, a larger molecule, the body's defences may be stimulated. A characteristic of the flea bite was that an initial nip would cause little trouble, but subsequent bites, after several days, would cause a strong skin reaction. For Feingold the way that haptens influence the immune response became a central interest. He noted that many of the chemicals used as drugs are of a similar size to the haptens in the flea's saliva and he began to wonder if adverse reactions to drugs reflected similar mechanisms.

Chemically, aspirin is known as acetylsalicylic acid and, like all drugs, has both desirable and undesirable features. In a few people the repeated taking of aspirin is associated with a slowly developing intolerance that eventually produces such a severe reaction that even death may result. A number of foods contain natural salicylates that are similar, although not identical, to aspirin. In people who are sensitive to aspirin, foods containing natural salicylates will induce the same type of adverse reaction. Table 6.2 lists foods that contain large and small amounts of natural salicylates. Foods such as almonds, tomatoes and cucumbers contain a high level of natural salicylates, as do a great many fruits, including apples, apricots, blackberries, cherries, currants, gooseberries, grapes, nectarines, oranges, peaches, plums, raspberries and strawberries. A diet was developed that avoided both aspirin and these foods, but some aspirin-sensitive patients still had adverse reactions. To what were they reacting?

Reports in the medical literature began to appear in which aspirin-sensitive patients reacted to the orange colouring agent tartrazine (E102, FD & C Yellow 5) often used in food, although the two chemicals were not of a similar structure. Feingold found that the reverse was also true: people sensitive to tartrazine also reacted to aspirin. Additives were added to the list of foods containing salicylates that were to be removed from the diet. At this time the research was still concerned with physical reactions to the diet, such as hives, rashes and asthmatic symptoms. The research had come a long way, but still had a long way to go.

In 1965 a woman in her early 40s went to the Kaiser-Permanente Medical Centre looking and feeling miserable. Her face was swollen, mainly around the eyes, and she had giant hives that were both painful and unsightly. Feingold wondered if artificial colours and flavours were responsible, and placed her on a diet

*Table 6.2* Foods to be eaten and avoided on the Feingold diet

---

*Eat foods low in salicylates*

---

Cereals and grains: barley, oats, rice, rye, wheat
Dairy: milk, cheese and eggs
Fruit: bananas, peeled pears
Fish and shellfish
Meat
Vegetables: beansprouts, brussels sprouts, cabbage, celery, leeks, lettuce,
    peas, peeled potatoes

---

*Do not eat foods high in salicylates*

---

Alcoholic drinks (other than gin and vodka)
Fruit juices
Most fruits
Most herbs and spices
Most nuts
Most processed foods
Most vegetables
Tomato sauce

---

that avoided these items. Within three days her skin condition had disappeared. Without her medical records, Feingold had no reason to suspect that this woman had a long record of aggressive behaviour. Only when her psychiatrist rang to ask about the treatment was it revealed that she had been undergoing psychotherapy for this problem for two years without success. Less than two weeks after she began an additive-free diet the woman's aggressive behaviour and the problems it caused for her family had disappeared. Both Feingold and the psychiatrist were extremely surprised. For the first time the adverse behavioural effect of additives was suspected. When the woman again attended the clinic her skin was normal and she reported that her behaviour had completely changed, except when she inadvertently ate food containing additives.

It is difficult to interpret such an observation, as many medical complaints spontaneously and inexplicably improve. When a doctor sees hundreds or thousands of patients, a spontaneous remission is going to occur by chance alone immediately after one of these consultations. How can the impact of the treatment be distinguished from simple coincidence?

Over the next years an increasing number of such observations were made: parents commented that when their children were treated for a physical symptom, their behavioural problems improved. Yet Feingold's primary interests were not behavioural, and he largely ignored these comments as curiosities. Then, in his late 60s, he underwent several operations and began to think seriously about retirement.

## Hyperactivity

During his convalescence Feingold began to hear about hyperkinesis-learning disabilities, also known as minimal brain dysfunction (damage) and by many parents as hyperactivity. In the early 1970s the media in the United States began to publicize several dozen scientific papers that were published over a short period. The message was simple: there was an alarming increase in the number of hyperactive children. As there was no precise definition of hyperactivity, the estimated numbers of affected children varied from 500,000 to 5 million. It seemed certain that the problem was increasing and reaching epidemic proportions. Paradoxically, the most common treatment, given to about 50 per cent of those so diagnosed, was daily medication with drugs that act in a manner similar to the stimulant amphetamine. The number of American children taking mind-altering drugs daily was measured in millions!

When Feingold had left paediatrics in 1945 to work on allergic problems, hyperactive children were few and far between. Twenty-five years later hyperactivity seemed to represent a major problem. In fact, many of the original estimates of the extent of the problem proved to be too high, although hyperactivity was still a matter of great concern in the United States in the early 1970s. What had changed over this period?

At the end of the Second World War artificial food colouring and flavouring were used to a very limited extent, but in the following decades their use increased progressively with the production of convenience foods. Thus there was circumstantial evidence to support the hypothesis that the increased use of additives caused hyperactivity in children. If we had drawn a graph showing the progressive increase in the incidence of hyperactivity and the increased use of food additives from 1945 to 1970, there would have been two parallel lines. The most such a graph suggests is that a hypothesis needs to be subjected to rigorous investigation; it is not in itself evidence that consuming additives is the cause of behavioural problems. Many things changed after the war: children progressively spent more time watching television; attitudes to child rearing became more liberal; single-parent families became more common. These factors, and many like them, offered possible explanations for the change in children's behaviour.

When Feingold began to discuss the possible influence of additives with friends and colleagues, word got out that he had a new explanation for the major social problem of hyperactivity. A television interview followed, the general public immediately accepted the idea and parents with problem children began to seek help. The first child that was seen by Feingold was typical of many. Johnny, aged 7, had a history of aggression and temper tantrums that could last for days. His mood swung from being wild and beyond control to extremely placid. His most worrying act had been to deliberately ride his tricycle into the path of an oncoming car. Routine blood and urine checks demonstrated no abnormality, and neurologically he was completely normal; physically he was well. Yet the prospect for a 7-year-old child was a daily dose of the stimulant drug Ritalin.

Instead, Johnny started the Feingold diet, avoiding foods containing natural salicylates and additives. For five months his mother kept a diary of his diet and behaviour. It included comments such as:

Chocolate bar at 11.30. Very noticeable behavior change at 2.30 p.m.

One teaspoon of antihistamine cough syrup at bedtime produced a raving maniac.[4]

The problem lasted for over twenty-four hours and was later interpreted as a reaction to the synthetic colours and flavours that are almost universally present in children's medicines.

Hamburger with relish. Juice punch. Super-charged behavior that lasts the next day.[5]

This was said to be a response to the natural salicylates in the fruit juice or in the cucumber in the relish.

This type of evidence was seen by Feingold as supporting the view that behaviour was being turned on and off by the food that was eaten. In many cases the use of the diet was found to remove the need for daily drugs. In 1973 and 1974 Feingold presented papers to the American Medical Association, which arranged press conferences that attracted journalists from around the world. The basic message was that between 40 and 70 per cent of hyperactive children who adhered to the Feingold diet demonstrated a marked reduction in hyperactive behaviour.

Yet when his findings were written up as scientific papers, and were submitted to the very prestigious *Journal of the American Medical Association*, they were rejected; later, his ideas were published in a less influential medical journal.[6] Feingold responded to the rejection of his peers by writing *Why Your Child Is Hyperactive*, in which he described his theory and findings for the general public. The book had a receptive market and Feingold Associations were formed in the United States, Canada, England, Australia, New Zealand, South Africa, Israel and Norway. These associations circulated information on the nature of additives in foods and acted as pressure groups demanding the removal of unnecessary food additives. In the year following the book's publication over 20,000 families were using the diet and over 100 Feingold Associations had been established throughout the world.

Why did the scientific community respond adversely to the Feingold hypothesis while so many parents found the ideas so attractive? It is easy to see why the parents of hyperactive children might find the theory convincing. As the children are so disruptive and emotionally draining, the parents are likely to be desperate, prepared to grasp at straws. Children's behaviour is particularly responsive to psychological factors and if a parent's belief in the diet creates the expectation that the child's behaviour will improve, in some cases this will happen.

The Feingold diet is so difficult to maintain in an absolute form that any behavioural lapse will often coincide with the recent consumption of a forbidden food. If no such lapse can be established, then it may be hypothesized that a food containing an additive undisclosed by the manufacturer has been eaten (there are many). Alternatively, the child may not have admitted eating commercially produced sweets or other items. These types of argument are unsatisfactory, although possibly superficially attractive. If the child's behaviour gets better, then it is due to the absence of additives; if the behaviour gets worse, then there must have been additives in the food, even though the evidence is lacking. If you can explain everything, then, effectively, you explain nothing. A good scientific theory must be falsifiable: it must be possible to disprove what is proposed.

For a scientist both the nature of the theory and the supporting evidence produce problems. The scientific community did not ignore Feingold, but found the anecdotal nature of his data, based on impressions rather than objective and systematic measures, unsatisfactory. The data lacked the characteristics of good scientific studies: there were no control groups, no one received a placebo, the procedure was not double-blind. As in each case the child, parent and doctor knew what was happening, subconsciously this may have influenced the situation. The history of drug evaluation is full of examples of compounds that appeared to work well when studied in an uncritical manner, but whose action completely disappeared when they were studied using rigorous methods. It was essential to establish whether in the case of the Feingold diet the reported improvements reflected the removal of additives, rather than the powerful and ubiquitous psychological response that occurs when a patient takes part in a research trial.

## The first scientific trial

Given the very reasonable concern that, in some individuals at least, the diet's beneficial effect may well be psychological, great attention was paid to the first attempt to test the hypothesis rigorously. The study was directed by Keith Conners, a psychologist then working at the University of Wisconsin. A sample of children who satisfied the criteria for the hyperactive syndrome were studied for a month. Measures of their behaviour, based on a range of psychological tests and ratings by their parents and teachers, were obtained. They were then randomly allocated to one of two diets: half had the Feingold diet and the other half another diet that also involved many changes in the food normally eaten. Parents and teachers agreed that both diets reduced the children's activity, and a few children were noted whose symptoms were markedly lower on the Feingold diet. Conners and his colleagues found that the behaviour of hyperactive children did not change in response to artificial food dyes, although there was some change on tests of attention.[7] The conclusion was that there might be a small subgroup of hyperactive children who benefited from the Feingold diet, but the results were inconclusive.

The validity of this study has been questioned.[8] The Conners study fed children specially baked biscuits that either did or did not contain a mixture of food dyes. A serious problem is that all the biscuits contained chocolate. As there is substantial evidence that chocolate is amongst the most common foods to which people react adversely, there is every reason to suggest that many of the children on both diets may have reacted to the chocolate. Thus it would be impossible to distinguish children who reacted to the chocolate from those who reacted to a mixture of additives and chocolate. The choice of the amount of additives has been criticized as being too low; when the level of additives consumed by American children was measured, it was found to be, on average, three times the level used by Conners, and some children consumed twelve times that amount.[9] Another cause for concern was that in the study the biscuits with additives were given twice on one day. In real life the additives would be consumed several times a day, every day for years on end, conditions under which it is more likely that a response would have occurred.

These criticisms cast substantial doubts on the reliability of Conners' conclusion. None the less, because Feingold offered little satisfactory scientific data, a great deal of attention was paid to Conners' findings. The Nutrition Foundation formed a National Advisory Committee on Hyperkinesis and Food Additives, which concluded that the studies to date:

have neither proven nor disproven the hypothesis that a diet free of artificial colors and flavors reduces the symptoms in a significant number of children with the hyperkinesis syndrome ... that data from critically designed and executed studies, free of the deficiencies of design noted, must be available before firm conclusions can be reached on the Feingold hypothesis.[10]

The question of additives and hyperactivity became a hot topic and research workers throughout the world raced each other to obtain relevant data. By 1983 a review of no fewer than twenty-three such studies was published. A statistical method was used to integrate the findings and it was concluded that 'diet modification is not an effective intervention for hyperactivity'.[11] When the findings were examined in terms of the approach taken, it was found that the more objective the measure of behaviour, the more likely it was that a negative finding would be found. Other extensive reviews of the literature drew similar conclusions, making comments such as 'the Feingold diet is probably not effective, except perhaps in a very small percentage of children'[12] and 'the broad conclusions were that his claims were probably exaggerated'.[13]

Bernard Rimland is the Director of the Institute for Child Behavior Research in San Diego, California, and has for many years articulately championed the view that many behavioural problems in children are a reflection of their diet. After surveying the reviews of the adequacy of Feingold's theory, he concluded that their negative assessments are 'unwarranted, probably incorrect, and very likely damaging'.[14]

In forthright style he dismissed the attempts to study Feingold over ten years as 'GIGO', computer jargon for garbage in, garbage out. If you carry out poor studies, then the results will necessarily be of little value. According to Rimland, the studies have simply failed to address the question. The Feingold diet aims to remove over 3,000 additives from the normal diet, yet most studies have examined fewer than ten dyes, often using doses much smaller than those commonly consumed. Yet, turning his argument on its head, there is no evidence that most of the thousands of additives do influence behaviour, although the possibility exists that in the future this will be demonstrated, in some cases at least.

What are we to conclude? Feingold's theory has to be taken seriously as the implications are widespread; there are few questions more important than the health of the next generation. Academics will be interested in discussing the minutiae of experiments, and may be happy to spend years running even more experiments, but parents concerned about their children, and policy makers dealing with the regulation of the food industry, need an answer. Even if the answer is not given with complete certainty there has to be some basis on which to proceed; the world cannot stand still.

As we will see, there is little doubt that some children react to food additives, although it is equally true that many unadulterated foods may also cause problems. However, the evidence that natural salicylates were important in this respect is very limited. The question is not 'Can food additives be the cause of problems?', but 'How frequently does this occur: is it an uncommon response or a major problem?'

The enormous difficulties associated with ensuring that every food item consumed by a hyperactive child is permitted by the Feingold diet means that almost certainly every child on the diet, on some occasion, eats a forbidden food. This is as true for children treated personally by Feingold as for those treated in later, more controlled studies. There is no reason to believe that all the children seen by Feingold himself systematically followed the diet to the last detail whereas children elsewhere did not. It follows that when Feingold finds substantial improvements in non-experimental situations whereas the phenomenon disappears or largely disappears in experimental situations, the only reasonable conclusion is that most of the improvement is psychological, a placebo response.

### *Food intolerance and hyperactivity*

Joseph Egger, a German paediatrician working in London, examined a related idea, that in at least some cases hyperactive behaviour was stimulated by some foods rather than additives. Migraine is defined as a severe headache that may be accompanied by nausea, vomiting and visual disturbances. In 1982–3 Egger and his colleagues studied the role of food in migraine at Great Ormond Street Hospital in London. They placed children on a diet consisting of one meat, one fruit, one vegetable and either rice or potatoes. After three to four weeks if the migraines had improved, other foods were systematically introduced. The results were remarkable: of eighty-eight children who completed the diet, seventy-eight recovered completely, and only six showed no improvement at all.[15] Perhaps these findings are not too surprising, as certain foods, such as chocolate, cheese, red wine and citrus fruit, are widely thought to trigger migraine attacks. (It is believed that they contain vasoactive amines that have a drug-like action on blood vessels.) Such a marked response did, however, require an elimination diet, as simply removing one food at a time was not associated with a similar beneficial response.

The major criticism of the Great Ormond Street study of migraine is that the children were so highly selected that they were not typical of those who have migraine. Most of them had many problems: hyperactivity, runny nose, diarrhoea, asthma, eczema or recurrent mouth ulcers. It is not usual for children who have migraine to display such a range of other problems. For this reason it is unclear if the findings can be generalized to most other children who have migraine.

That the children had symptoms other than migraine had an unexpected advantage, as it was noticed that the behaviour of some children also improved; they became less active.[16] In some cases the food that produced migraine was not the same as that which caused hyperactivity. Later, Egger and his colleagues followed up this chance observation by systematically examining the impact of food on hyperactive children.[17]

The children studied were about 7 years old and had a history of short attention span, distractability and over-activity for at least a year. A high proportion of the children suffered with allergic-like problems: 71 per cent reported abdominal discomfort, 43 per cent a chronic runny nose, 37 per cent had skin rashes and 63 per cent had headaches. Initially, the children were placed on an oligoantigenic diet – one that consisted of only a few food items that are unlikely to cause problems of food intolerance. A typical diet consisted of lamb, chicken, potatoes, rice, banana, apple, any brassica, water, and multi-vitamin and calcium tablets.

If the parents thought that the child improved, the next stage was started, in which other foods were gradually reintroduced. One at a time additional foods were introduced each day for a week. If the symptoms returned, the food was withdrawn from the diet; if not, then the food was maintained in the diet. The possibility that the child responded to the orange colourant tartrazine (E102) and the preservative benzoic acid was examined. First it was established that the child had no adverse reaction to oranges or sugar, and then orange squash that contained the fruit, sugar, tartrazine and benzoic acid was introduced.

The long procedure was not yet finished. The possibility that the reaction was a placebo response had to be considered. Pairs of foods were prepared that appeared to be similar, although one contained a problem food and the other did not. One recipe might contain cow's milk and the other goat's or soya milk; one wheat, the other rice or oats; one orange juice, the other pineapple juice. Tartrazine and benzoic acid or a placebo were given in capsules. Each day the parents gave one of these specially prepared foods to their child without knowing if it contained the problem food or the placebo. Each day the severity of the child's symptoms was rated. The findings were clear-cut. The behaviour of the children was significantly better when they did not receive the foods that were a problem for them. Most of the physical symptoms, such as abdominal pains and runny noses, also improved.

The commonest items causing adverse reactions were benzoic acid and tartrazine (79 per cent of cases), but no child reacted to these alone, and no fewer than forty-six foods were found to cause a reaction in at least some children. In addition, 6.5 per cent of those

*Table 6.3* **Foodstuffs to which allergic children react hyperactively**

| Foodstuffs | Children reacting (%) | Foodstuffs | Children reacting (%) |
|---|---|---|---|
| Colorants and preservatives | 79 | Ham/bacon | 20 |
| | | Pineapple | 19 |
| Cow's milk | 64 | Sugar | 16 |
| Chocolate | 59 | Beef | 16 |
| Grapes | 49 | Beans | 15 |
| Wheat | 49 | Peas | 15 |
| Oranges | 45 | Malt | 15 |
| Cow's-milk cheese | 40 | Apples | 13 |
| Hen's egg | 39 | Pork | 13 |
| Peanuts | 32 | Pears | 12 |
| Maize | 29 | Chicken | 11 |
| Fish | 23 | Potatoes | 11 |
| Oats | 23 | Tea | 10 |
| Melons | 21 | Coffee | 10 |
| Tomatoes | 20 | Other nuts | 10 |

Only foods to which more than 10 per cent of children reacted are included. There are other foods that stimulated a response in less than 10 per cent of cases.

*Source:* Egger *et al.*, *Lancet*, 14, 1985, 540–45.

studied responded to pollen, house-dust or perfume. Table 6.3 gives a list of the food items found by Egger to most commonly provoke hyperactivity. The presence of items such as milk, chocolate, wheat, cheese and some fruit shows the range of possible problem foods. While the careful design of the study by Egger and his co-workers means that we must take very seriously the suggestion that diet can contribute to the behavioural problems of children, the results need to be placed in perspective: although 82 per cent of children showed some improvement when their problem foods were eliminated from their diet, only 27 per cent improved completely.

The picture suggested by these data is very different from Feingold's hypothesis. Feingold proposed that the problem was caused by a group of food items having in common a single action similar to an adverse reaction to aspirin. In contrast, Egger found an adverse reaction to many foods, most of which are not chemically related to salicylates, and which have no known pharmacological action. Some of the foods that are problem items in the Feingold diet, for example peaches and cucumbers, were very low in the list of problem foods in Egger's study. Equally, other foods, for example chocolate, that had been part of the placebo in some studies of the Feingold diet were found to be a frequent cause of problems in Egger's trials.

Great care should be taken in generalizing the findings of the Egger study. The children who were found to react to such a range of foods were very highly selected. They were a minority of the minority of children that display hyperactive symptoms: they were selected for being severely overactive, and many displayed the physical symptoms of allergic reactions. There is evidence, however, that children who display hyperactivity are more likely to have a history of classic allergic problems such as asthma or eczema as well as being more likely to be food intolerant.[18]

Many questions remain. For example, it is known that allergic reactions to various items can interact. It would be interesting to examine the impact of food on hyperactivity at different times of the year, when hay fever is and is not a problem. It is simply not known whether the allergic reaction to food directly influences the brain or whether hyperactivity is a psychological response to the stress of the allergy. It is similarly not known how many children who do not have a history of allergic reactions react to food by becoming hyperactive. However, research at the Institute of Child Health and Institute of Psychiatry in London has found similar effects to those in Egger's findings, although less marked, in children more typical of the normal range of hyperactive children.[19]

## *Final comments*

While the weight of evidence supports the view that the vast majority of hyperactive children will not benefit from Feingold's diet, it should be remembered that a minority of children do react adversely to aspects of their diet. Placed in the context of many other suggested causes of hyperactivity (Table 6.4), there is no reason to believe that diet-related factors are of significance in many cases.

*Table 6. 4* **Suggested causes of hyperactivity**

---

Brain damage
Brain dysfunction
Drug-taking during pregnancy
Emotional insecurity
Epilepsy
Food intolerance
Genetic factors
Lead poisoning
Maternal smoking
Psycho-social conditions
Sensitivity to food additives

---

A dietary approach to hyperactivity should not be lightly suggested, as it requires an abrupt and substantial change in lifestyle. Children on this kind of restricted diet are unable to eat meals provided by schools and restaurants, and are not able to eat commercially produced confectionery; parents must exercise continuing vigilance while shopping and preparing food. The diet may easily set hyperactive children apart from their peers when their behavioural history will have already caused problems. In some, but not all, cases there have been suggestions that such a restricted diet is the cause of deficiencies of vitamins and other micronutrients. More seriously, on rare occasions anaphylactic shock may result when food is reintroduced, with the possibility of fatal consequences.

Some scientists have been extremely critical of Feingold, raising the ethical question of prematurely exposing the general public to a largely unexamined hypothesis. An Australian doctor, whose opinion is representative of this position, commented, 'I personally feel there is no greater breach of medical ethics than that of foisting a potentially worthless or dangerous treatment on a credulous public. Theirs may be the right to believe in magic and panaceas but ours as a profession is to act responsibly, cautiously, and scientifically, though not prejudicially.'

Such a view may seem rather harsh. Feingold believed that he had discovered a possible cause for a rapidly increasing and very worrying problem, although he seemed unaware of the weakness of the data on which his views rested. Rather than being subjected to a hard sell, the response of the public reflected the heart-felt need of people worried about their children's future, while being subjected to the extreme emotional stress of living with a hyperactive child.

This episode illustrates several aspects of the study of nutrition and behaviour. People have a ready appetite for messages that suggest simple nutritional solutions to worrying behavioural problems. There is every reason to believe that any widely discussed effect of a change in diet will be widely taken up, a phenomenon that gives researchers a responsibility to be cautious in making recommendations. Any unjustified recommendation will give false hope and prevent the following of alternative approaches that are known to be beneficial. Psychological complaints are extremely susceptible to placebo effects – if you give people reason to believe that they will improve, then in many cases there will be a significant change for the better. However, irrespective of the scientific evidence, it is likely that the parents of children whose lives appear to have been transformed by a change of diet will hold Feingold's theory in the highest regard.

For a scientist the most rigorous experiments are required before you can conclude that a nutritional manipulation is beneficial. To the extent that subsequent research has supported the idea that at least tartrazine and benzoic acid can be a source of problems in some children, Feinberg was partially correct, although it seems likely that it is a minority of hyperactive children for whom diet is a problem. There is almost no evidence that it is useful to remove a wide range of food items containing natural salicylates from the diet. It seems improbable that general dietary advice can usefully be offered to the parents of hyperactive children; where there is an adverse response to food items, it will differ from child to child. The existence and nature of any particular child's dietary problem will be definitely established only by the most rigorous studies.

# CHAPTER 7

# Glucose: the Food of the Brain

## Sugar gets a bad press

When it comes to concerns that diet may influence our behaviour, sugar competes with additives as the item most likely to be the source of worry. One of a long series of popular books that have discussed the impact of sugar in the diet began, 'For one person in every ten, sugar is a deadly food, paving the way towards a hundred distressing physical symptoms, plus all the tortures of neurotic and even psychotic symptoms.'[1] One psychologist described sugar as 'the most ubiquitous toxin'.[2] Particularly in the United States, there is a widespread belief that sugar causes behavioural problems in children. Does sugar deserve such a bad press?

There are three ways in which sugar has been said to influence behaviour. Firstly, consuming too much sugar has been said to deprive the body of vitamins and minerals. This is the familiar argument that sugar offers only 'empty calories', which provide energy, but, because it is so refined during manufacture, fails to offer an adequate source of vitamins (see Chapters 4 and 9). Sugar is, of course, only one of many highly refined foods from which minerals and vitamins have been removed. Secondly, it is known that a minority of the population lacks the ability to digest sugar, and that this food intolerance is associated with changes in behaviour (see Chapter 5). Thirdly, it has been suggested that sugar causes swings in blood glucose levels. After we have eaten, as the food is digested, glucose is released into the bloodstream. It has been proposed that eating sugar causes a particularly large and rapid rise in the level of glucose in the blood, which after a few hours falls to a level that disrupts the functioning of the brain.

There is some truth in each of these three ideas. The first two are dealt with elsewhere in this book: this chapter examines the impact of the levels of glucose in blood (blood glucose) and the role played by sugar in the diet in influencing them.

## Who eats sugar?

Who eats sugar? The answer is we all do, most of us in very large quantities. There are two major groups of sugars. The first are the monosaccharides, or simple sugars, of which glucose and fructose are examples. Most carbohydrates in food are converted into glucose during digestion, and fructose is the sugar in fruit. The second group of sugars is the disaccharides, which consist of two monosaccharides linked together. The sugar in our sugar bowl is sucrose, a chemical combination of glucose and fructose. Here we will use 'sugar' to refer to sucrose, and 'sugars' to refer generically to all simple and complex sugars. It should, however, be remembered that, when necessary, protein and fat, and not only sugars, can be converted into glucose and raise the levels in the blood.

Carbohydrates, that is sugars and starches, are, apart from water, the single largest item in the diet of most individuals. However, in recent years the consumption of carbohydrate has declined in industrialized societies while the consumption of sugar has increased. Figure 7.1 shows the steady increase in the consumption of sugar over the last 250 years in the United Kingdom: only rationing during the two world wars produced a temporary halt to the increase.[3] Two hundred years ago the British consumed 1.8–2.3 kg (4–5 lb) of sugar each a year. By 1850 this had risen to about 11 kg (25 lb) and today it is about 45 kg (100 lb) a year. The British now eat as much sugar in a week as they used to eat in six months. Most Britons would deny that they eat about 142 g (5 oz) of sugar a day, but, as this is an average, there are many who eat substantially more.

It is easy to see how such figures could arise: eating a sweetened breakfast cereal with added sugar; adding sugar to several cups

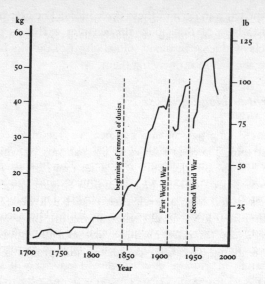

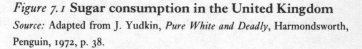

*Figure 7.1* **Sugar consumption in the United Kingdom**
*Source:* Adapted from J. Yudkin, *Pure White and Deadly*, Harmondsworth, Penguin, 1972, p. 38.

of tea or coffee during the day; eating cakes, biscuits, chocolate, other confectionery and sweetened desserts. The consumption of fizzy drinks can increase markedly the intake of sugar: a 100 ml can of cola contains 10 g of sugar. The average American drinks more than 300 cans of such drinks a year: Coca-Cola is the world's single largest user of sugar. It is only too easy to consume large quantities of sugar.

Figure 7.1 shows that the consumption of sugar has apparently declined in recent years. In part this may reflect people's concern about health and, in particular, obesity. However, if you add the consumption of sugar to the other sweet compounds used in food manufacture, such as high-fructose syrup, then total consumption has changed little. The food industry uses a great deal of sugar, but we are often unaware of its presence in the foods we eat. It may be hidden in such unlikely items as tomato ketchup, canned peas and baked beans. The cheapness of sugar, its attractive taste and its ability to preserve food make it widely used by the food industry.

## *The control of blood glucose*

Within thirty minutes of a person eating a meal a surge of glucose enters the bloodstream. There is a series of mechanisms by which the body tries to keep blood glucose within a set range of 70–100 milligrams of glucose per decilitre blood (mg/dl) (Figure 7.2). If blood glucose rises to too high a level, then tissues dehydrate. If blood glucose falls to too low a level (below 40 mg/dl), the symptoms of hypoglycaemia (literally meaning low glucose) appear. These include trembling, sweating, confusion and problems of perception.

After a meal nearly all the carbohydrate absorbed from the gut circulates in the blood as glucose. The blood glucose rises rapidly, so the body needs to bring it back within the optimal range. The

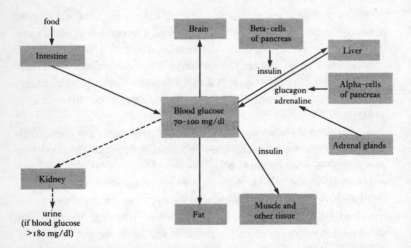

*Figure 7.2* **Control of blood glucose**

pancreas produces insulin, which stimulates the liver to store glucose in the form of glycogen and speeds the entry of glucose into cells. Both mechanisms cause the level of glucose in the blood to fall. An inability of the pancreas to produce insulin results in diabetes mellitus; without an adequate release of insulin, blood glucose remains high.

The pancreas also secretes a second hormone, glucagon, which acts in the opposite way to insulin. When the blood glucose level falls, glucagon enters the bloodstream and causes the liver to release stored glucose. A very low level of blood glucose causes the release of a third hormone, adrenaline, which also stimulates the release of stored glucose from the liver.

Although the brain represents only 2 per cent of body weight, it uses 20 to 30 per cent of the whole body's energy. Strangely, the energy stores in the brain are extremely small when compared with the high rate with which energy is used. If they are not replenished, the stores will be used up in under ten minutes. The brain is unusual in that under normal circumstances it uses glucose exclusively as a source of fuel. The high activity of the brain suggests that we should consider the possibility that it may be sensitive to the provision of glucose.

## Can you handle glucose?

The Glucose Tolerance Test examines the body's ability to control the level of glucose in the blood. It is most likely to be used by the medical profession to diagnose diabetes, some forms of liver disorder and only rarely food-stimulated hypoglycaemia. Initially, a baseline blood glucose value is measured in an individual who has fasted overnight and has not eaten breakfast. A drink containing glucose is administered and the glucose level in the blood is monitored, for three hours in the case of diabetes, and longer in the case of suspected food-induced hypoglycaemia (Figure 7.3).

There is no such thing as a normal response in a glucose tolerance test, as, within limits, healthy people can differ in their response. Blood glucose will rise by about 50 per cent during the first hour after the drink; it will approach the fasting value around

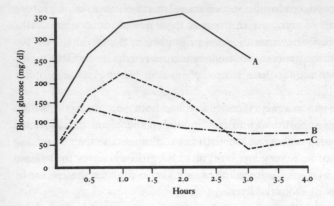

*Figure 7.3* **Glucose Tolerance Test**

After fasting overnight a drink containing 50 g of glucose is drunk
and blood glucose levels are monitored for several hours. The way
that curve A rises to, and stays at, high levels, is characteristic of a
diabetic. Curve B rises and returns to its baseline within two hours
and does not indicate any problems. Curve C rises to high values and
then falls rapidly to levels lower than its baseline. Being less than 40
mg/dl it can be described as characteristic of hypoglycaemia.

the second hour; it will then in some, but not all, cases fall below
fasting values. After we eat, the glucose levels in the blood rise until
they stimulate the pancreas to produce insulin, the hormone that
causes glucose values to level out and eventually fall (Figure 7.3).
Depending on the size and duration of the insulin response, the
individual may end up with blood glucose values less than the
fasting levels.

There have been many suggestions that the tendency to develop low blood glucose levels may be associated with changes in
behaviour, in particular irritability (see Chapter 8). It is said that
some individuals react to a meal containing sugar by releasing such
large amounts of insulin that after several hours blood glucose falls
to levels that are described as hypoglycaemic. In fact, it was only
with the discovery of diabetes that the possibility of a food-induced
hypoglycaemic response was suspected: if the production of too

little insulin in diabetes was associated with high levels of blood glucose, was it possible that the release of too much insulin might result in low levels of blood glucose?

## Food-induced hypoglycaemia

The people most familiar with hypoglycaemia are diabetics, who sooner or later may take too much insulin, so that their blood glucose falls to a level that prevents the normal functioning of the brain. At first they feel hungry, weak and anxious, and may have palpitations and begin to sweat. They feel faint, dizzy, have a severe headache and start to shake. These are the first symptoms of hypoglycaemia. If glucose values fall further, a lack of fuel disrupts the functioning of the brain; confusion, blurred vision, slurred and non-sensical speech, amnesia and bizarre behaviour result. If low glucose levels persist, coma and even death can result. There is evidence that repeated coma induced by low blood glucose levels results in brain damage.[4]

In 1924 Searle Harris, an American doctor, described spontaneous, reactive or food-induced hypoglycaemia.[5] He had observed five non-diabetic patients with symptoms similar to those that result from insulin-induced hypoglycaemia. The first was another physician, who complained that one hour before his midday meal he felt 'weak, nervous and so hungry that he could not work.'

Rather than being due to a lack of food, these symptoms reflected the production of too much insulin. The solution was easy; eating five smaller meals at regular intervals during the day made the problem disappear.

### How common is it?

Because eating sugar very rapidly raises blood glucose levels, and hence the release of insulin, it has been assumed in many popular books that a diet high in sugar is likely to be associated with a tendency to develop the symptoms of hypoglycaemia. There is, however, a marked contrast between the frequency with which popular writers and many clinicians suggest that hypoglycaemia occurs. One popular book claimed that hypoglycaemia caused by too much sugar in the diet was a problem for one person in ten.[6] In contrast a medical text commented that reactive hypoglycaemia 'was uncommon'.[7] Who is correct?

For the medical profession the criteria required for a diagnosis of hypoglycaemia are that blood glucose levels are below 40 mg/dl; there are characteristic symptoms, such as sweating and feeling anxious; the symptoms appear two to three hours after eating; the symptoms disappear if food is consumed. Even in a Glucose Tolerance Test very low blood glucose levels are not common. In an extensive study of 650 normal subjects the lowest blood glucose was on average 65 mg/dl.[8] Only 2.5 per cent reached values that would have allowed hypoglycaemia to be diagnosed. The Glucose Tolerance Test is, however, an unusual situation. How many people fast overnight, then consume 50 g of glucose without any protein, fat or starch, and then do not eat again for four or five hours? It is a grossly unnatural procedure. It may be a valuable way of diagnosing diabetes, but it is of little use for assessing the reaction to food. Yet it is the evidence from this procedure on which the claims that sugar in the diet produces psychological problems are based.

In contrast, everyday changes in blood glucose have been little studied. For example, when nineteen individuals eating normally were monitored, 'very little variation in glucose concentrations during the day' was observed.[9] This is quite different from the results obtained using a Glucose Tolerance Test. A clear picture emerges. When normally fed healthy subjects are studied, their glucose levels tend to be stable. Glucose values rise after a meal but typically return to levels well above those required to diagnose hypoglycaemia. In normal individuals, fed in a usual manner, a hypoglycaemic response is uncommon. In fact, a diagnosis of reactive hypoglycemia is best achieved by the use of a Meal Tolerance Test, in which sugar is combined with fat and protein, which help to prevent marked changes in blood glucose levels.

There is no doubt that some people react to their diet by becoming hypoglycaemic, although in the vast majority of the population it is uncommon following a normal meal. It is, however, relatively easy to induce a marked swing in blood glucose levels with an appropriate, yet unlikely, diet. Consuming glucose and alcohol would be one example. Alcohol increases the ability of glucose to stimulate the release of insulin from the pancreas. An alcoholic lunch followed by a chocolate bar is not to be recommended. The resulting high levels of insulin will result in low blood glucose levels several hours later.

### Dealing with food-induced hypoglycaemia

If you think you may have reactive hypoglycaemia, what should you do? Taking a lump of sugar or a drink containing sugar will have a marked effect. Within a few minutes both the physical and psychological symptoms will disappear. However, the benefits will be short-lived, as the rapid increase in blood glucose will be followed by a rapid decrease. The ideal solution is to prevent rapid swings in blood glucose by eating foods that are only slowly released into the bloodstream. Paradoxically, the way to avoid reactive hypoglycaemia is to avoid sugar in the diet and to eat small meals at regular intervals.

### *Blood glucose and mood*

Few of us will have experienced the mental and emotional symptoms of food-induced hypoglycaemia. Many, however, will have responded to feeling tired and a little low, perhaps in the late afternoon, by eating a biscuit or a chocolate bar. In doing this we are assuming that the resulting rise in blood glucose will give us a mental boost. Is there evidence that blood glucose levels, not low enough to induce hypoglycaemic symptoms, but lower than optimal, produce mild psychological problems? Does that biscuit in the afternoon improve your mood?

It seems that it depends on what you have been doing. If we simply measure blood glucose and measure mood, we find that there is a relationship, but it is very small. Blood glucose levels are not the major determinant of mood. People with higher blood glucose levels report themselves as slightly more relaxed yet energetic; those with lower levels as slightly more tense and tired.[10] Although this association has been reported on several occasions, blood glucose accounts for only a few per cent in the variation in mood. This conclusion may conflict with the subjective feelings of many of us who, when we feel tired and irritable in the late afternoon, find that a meal revives us.

This difference may reflect the situation in which mood and blood glucose have been studied. When mood and blood glucose levels have been found to have little if any relationship, people have been sitting around doing very little. It seems clear that under these conditions increasing blood glucose levels is not going to markedly improve your mood; other factors are likely to predominate. In contrast, if blood glucose levels are raised while people are performing a demanding task, there is a tendency for them to feel more alert for a longer period.[11] Increasing blood glucose levels does not make people feel more energetic, but it can prevent them feeling tired when they have been under pressure.

## *Does high blood glucose keep us going longer?*

Is it only mood that is influenced by the increases in blood glucose that follow a meal? Workers in a forge in Lancashire, who started work at 7.45am, usually went to work without breakfast, and first ate during a mid-morning break at 10.00am. The forging of metal is a hot, noisy, dusty job that takes place in air full of noxious fumes. First thing in the morning workers received either a glucose or a low energy drink. Any accident that occurred had to be recorded in the factory accident book; they varied from abrasions to broken bones.[12] Figure 7.4 shows a clear picture. More accidents took place in the morning, when most workers had not eaten breakfast and their daily body rhythm is associated with lower efficiency. However, those who had drunk a glucose drink were less likely to have suffered an accident.

Working in a forge involves heavy manual work. It is easy to

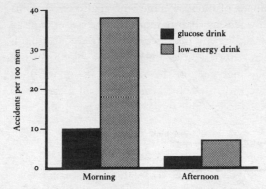

*Figure 7.4* **A glucose drink decreases accidents at work**
Workers in a forge were less likely to have an accident if they had a
glucose drink first thing in the morning.
*Source:* Data from Brooke *et al.*, *Scandinavian Journal of Work and*
*Environmental Health*, 6, 1980, 66–72.

believe that a shortage of blood glucose may limit the ability to
perform manual work and hence increase the likelihood of an accident. However, is there also a problem for those of us who do not
carry out manual work?

One situation in which we are required to concentrate for long
periods is driving. Clearly, any study of driving has the potential to
disturb the driver and cause an accident. One solution is to use a
driving simulator that has the controls of a normal car. The task is
to follow a road, projected on to a screen, that changes at a speed
that depends on how much the accelerator is depressed. German
researchers monitored driving in a simulator that covered 110 kilometres of winding road and took about 70 minutes. The number of
times the line in the centre of the road was crossed, the number of
times the 'car' crashed and the number of gear-changes were recorded. Performance was compared when the drivers did, and did
not, have a glucose drink. As the distance driven increased, so did
the number of errors (Figure 7.5). There was little difference for the
first 70 kilometres, but after 110 kilometres, the driving of those
who had drunk the glucose drink was significantly better.[13] These

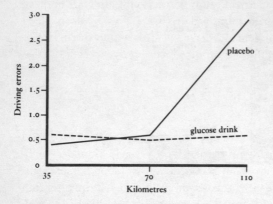

*Figure 7.5* **A glucose drink decreases errors while driving**
The number of errors while driving in a simulator was lower after taking a glucose drink.
*Source:* Keul *et al.*, *Aktuelle Ernährungsmedizin*, 7, 1982, 7–14.

and similar laboratory tests support the view that food-induced increases in blood glucose levels will help us to maintain our level of concentration over a period of time.

A doctor in a hospital accident unit in North Wales noted that he had seen several lorry drivers who, for no apparent reason, had crashed across the central reservation of a motorway. When the blood glucose levels of these drivers had been measured, they had proved to be extremely low.[14] Many lorry drivers start work early in the morning to avoid the traffic and leave home without breakfast. Although road traffic accidents occur for many reasons, it is possible that a low blood glucose level might be one predisposing factor. In Chapter 12 the ability of a glucose-containing drink to remove the negative effect of not eating breakfast will be described.

The physical effort of driving is small compared with manual work, yet a drink containing glucose still improved performance.[15] It is perhaps not so surprising that driving, which may require intense concentration for several hours, might benefit from the provision of glucose. Remember that the brain uses 20 to 30 per cent of the body's energy supplies, and has relatively small stores of glucose, its basic fuel. In the German study it was only after an hour of driving that a glucose drink improved driving. It seems reasonable to suggest that only when demands have been placed on the brain for a long period will the ability to supply glucose prove to be limited.

## We are not all the same

Not everybody responds similarly to a particular level of blood glucose. Generally, the symptoms of hypoglycaemia appear when the blood glucose falls to about 40 mg/dl. When blood glucose is in the range 40–50 mg/dl, performance on tasks that require attention tends to be disrupted. There are, however, large individual differences. The ability of some people to perform psychological tasks can be disrupted by blood glucose as high as 70 mg/dl, whereas in others even blood glucose below 40 mg/dl is not disruptive. Although the origin of these individual differences is unknown, if food relieves the symptoms of hypoglycaemia, functioning tends to be disrupted when glucose levels are at higher levels.[16]

## Sugar and hyperactive children

So widespread is the assumption in the United States that sugar causes behavioural problems in children, that a single advertisement in a newspaper, asking for children who react adversely to sugar, produces responses from dozens of parents. The parents hope that taking part in a scientific study dealing with sugar will show them how to improve the behaviour of their child. A mother wrote concerning her son's behaviour:

Tom, my 4-year-old, is usually a happy and pleasant child, who plays well with his older sister. He is able to concentrate for long periods on children's television programs. At an early age I found that if I gave him chocolate, or other sweets that contained high levels of sugar, then his personality changed. He starts running wildly around the house, torments his sister and the family dog to the extent that I am worried that the dog is going to injure him. This reaction occurs within minutes and lasts for over an hour. It is only after sugar snacks that I have seen this reaction.[17]

Many of the early suggestions that children respond adversely to sugar reflected clinical observations. William Crook, an American paediatrician, was convinced that sucrose is a leading cause of hyperactivity.[18] His conviction owed much to his experience as a clinician. When sugar was removed from the diet of hyperactive children, their behaviour improved; when sugar was reintroduced into the diet, the symptoms rapidly reappeared. Faced with such evidence, it is easy to see why people would be convinced that sugar was responsible for the children's problems. In fact, all we have is a very good example of the need for well-controlled scientific studies. For the clinician it does not matter that both the parents and children know that sugar is being removed from the diet and that they believe it will improve the children's behaviour. In contrast, the scientist needs to establish that any behavioural improvement is a response to sugar, rather than to psychological factors such as expectation or suggestion.

The examination of the diet of hyperactive children gave another early impetus to the view that sugar was inducing behavioural problems. A group of twenty-eight hyperactive children was recruited following newspaper, radio and television announcements.[19] The group was compared with children who were chosen to be as similar as possible, except they did not have behavioural problems. The parents of all the children were asked to keep a diary of the food eaten for seven days. From these data estimates were made of the consumption of sugar.

The behaviour of these children was videotaped and categorized by observers unaware of the purpose of the study. Within the groups there were different relationships between diet and behaviour. In the hyperactive children there was a correlation between sugar consumption and destructive or aggressive behaviour (hitting, kicking or throwing items), although the same dietary measure did not relate to activity. The opposite picture emerged with the control group, where there was a significant correlation between sugar intake and activity, but none to aggressive behaviour.

Another study related the diet of 4–5-year-old children who were not hyperactive to their ability to sustain attention.[20] These children were eating as much as 40 per cent of their calories as refined sugar. Those whose sugar intake was in the top 25 per cent were less able to sustain attention than those in the bottom 25 per cent. The pattern of sugar consumption seemed to be fairly stable; it appeared that a dietary pattern had become established in early life.

All the problems of a correlational approach apply to these findings. Did the sugar intake influence the behaviour? Did the behaviour influence the sugar intake? Did some third factor influence both attention and sugar intake? For example, the mothers of children with a high sugar intake were said to be less likely to have rules concerning access to foods. The impulsive nature of the hyperactive child may have made it more difficult for them to prevent themselves eating pleasant-tasting items.

Accepting the problems inherent with this type of approach, the findings could not be readily dismissed. It needed to be established if changing the amount of sugar in children's diet did or did not change their behaviour.

### Challenging children with sugar

A number of attempts were then made to give children sugar while monitoring their behaviour. The responses were not straightforward. With preschool children, a drink containing sugar increased activity and decreased the time spent attending to the task in hand.[21] The picture with older children was different. The activity of children on a psychiatric ward decreased when they were challenged with sugar.[22] In a similar study, 10-year-old boys whose parents thought that they responded adversely to dietary sugar were monitored. Again, they responded to sugar with a slight decrease in activity, although tests of memory and attention were unaffected.[23] Rather than demonstrating that sugar increases activity, with these older children the opposite was the case: they became less active. There is no evidence that sugar is a universal problem for children.

A fourth study graphically illustrates the importance of relying only on well-designed experiments when examining the impact of diet.[24] Sixteen children (average age 6.8 years) whose parents felt that sugar caused adverse reactions were monitored. In the first part of the study nine of the children reacted adversely when given a candy bar to eat. They responded to the candy bar in the manner that their parents predicted: they became more active and their behaviour deteriorated. However, when their response to sugar was examined in a double-blind trial 'the prevalence of adverse sugar reaction in this group was zero . . .'[25]

This study very clearly illustrates the need for well-controlled trials. The expectations of both the children and the parents are extremely important. An idea becomes rooted in the minds of both the children and the parents: sugar will produce adverse behaviour. Such an idea can easily become a self-fulfilling prophecy. When parents teach children that they will behave badly if they eat sugar, when they do eat sugar, they act in the way that their parents expect. Equally, the expectation that the removal of sugar will improve the situation may give a psychological lift. The feeling is created that the cause of the disruptive behaviour has been eliminated; for psychological reasons the child's behaviour improves.

It is difficult to overstate the importance of the observation that children's behaviour was disrupted when they knowingly ate a candy bar but that it was not when they received sugar in double-blind conditions. The adverse response to sugar, and other food-related items such as additives, in many cases is psychological. When children respond to their diet, there are two possible explanations. Firstly, that physiologically they respond to a food item in a negative manner. Secondly, that their parents have taught them to respond negatively to the food. Both are possible, although the weight of evidence is that the response is more often psychological rather than physiological in origin.

## A paradox

Innumerable books and media articles have alerted the population to the possibility, if not the probability, that negative responses to food items may occur. The anxiety that has been generated in parents has led them to pay great attention to their children's diet. They have created the exact problem about which these articles were warning. Initially, in most children there is no adverse biological response to sugar, but the parents' concern teaches children to respond negatively. It turns out that the books with the scare stories about children's diet are partially correct because they have helped to create the problem that they were trying to prevent.

### Are there really sugar-reactive children?

In concluding that a child's adverse response to sugar is more likely to be psychological than physiological in nature, it should be remembered that some children do respond adversely to sugar. One problem of taking evidence only from double-blind studies as conclusive proof is that you can ignore the individual who reacts in an unusual way. The conclusion that most hyperactive children are not displaying an adverse reaction to sugar is unavoidable. A conclusion that no child reacts adversely to sugar would be misleading.

When you are dealing with rare events, the evidence of case studies becomes critical. In blind tests a hyperactive boy and his mother responded to sugar by becoming irritable and hyperactive, and by developing headaches.[26] The significance of this type of clinical observation is difficult to evaluate. Even with blind controls, it is impossible to establish whether such a response to sugar is extremely rare or commonplace. When discussing sugar in this context it should be remembered that many other foods, including milk, wheat, egg, cocoa and corn, cause similar problems (see Chapters 5 and 6).

When sugar, milk, wheat, egg, cocoa and corn were removed from the diets of hyperactive children, some improvement was observed in twelve out of twenty-three cases.[27] When sugar was subsequently replaced in the diet, seven out of twenty-one reported increased hyperactivity. This was not specifically related to sugar: it also applied in four cases with cocoa, five with corn and six with milk. The picture that emerged was of a sample of children who reacted to many aspects of the diet, and even more commonly to dust and pollen than to food. There was no suggestion that sugar was the predominant or exclusive problem.

## Artificial sweeteners

One response to concerns about eating too much sugar is to use an artificial sweetener. These products offer a pleasantly sweet taste but lack the calories, and hopefully any other negative characteristics, of sugar. As luck would have it, artificial sweeteners, such as aspartame, have, in turn, become a cause for concern.

Frank's mother had started to become concerned about him becoming overweight and changed his usual fruit squash to a low-calorie product. During a hot summer Frank drank the new squash throughout the day. Over a period of two weeks he became increasingly angry and frustrated. He burst into tears and displayed violent outbursts. Finally, there was a hyperactive episode when he threw things around his bedroom, and lay screaming, kicking and thumping the floor. The dramatic episode resulted in Frank seeing a paediatrician, who explored recent changes in Frank's routine, trying to explain his remarkable change in behaviour. Perhaps because there was no obvious alternative, it was suggested that the change in drink might be the problem.

Frank's mother was less than convinced by this explanation; a low-calorie drink seemed a benign, healthy product, not something that changed personality. On the basis that there was little to lose, she again bought the original sugar-containing drink. Frank returned to being an affectionate, loving 4-year-old. Having something of the scientist in her, and not being convinced that the change was more than coincidence, after some weeks she bought the low-calorie drink again. This time within thirty minutes Frank had a violent headache and became more aggressive than on previous occasions. The low-calorie drink contained aspartame as the sweetener. From then on Frank's mother avoided products containing this sweetener and such extremes of behaviour have not recurred.

Although Frank's case is more convincing than many clinical reports, you cannot exclude the possibility that the response was psychological. Although Frank's family assumed that aspartame caused the problem, a fruit drink is a cocktail of many chemicals. You could not be certain that the sweetener was to blame.

Before being approved for use in the United States, aspartame went through a turbulent period. There had been concern, based on animal studies, that it might cause brain damage. Animals receiving aspartame had been said to be more susceptible to seizures. Questions had been raised about the quality of some of the scientific research on which the claim that it was safe was based. In the United States the Federal Food and Drug Administration withheld its approval of aspartame on several occasions. The debate was entirely about the possibility that it might induce cancer or cause brain damage; the possibility that behaviour might be adversely influenced was not considered. It took nearly twenty years for Searle Pharmaceuticals to gain approval, in 1981, for the use of aspartame in the United States.

There have been attempts to compare the behaviour of groups of children who on different occasions have drinks containing sugar, aspartame or neither of these. With preschool children, no differences in activity were found after the three drinks.[28] In other studies some minor complaints have been related to the taking of aspartame, but if there are effects, they are subtle in nature, nothing like Frank's reaction.

Was Frank's reaction to the drink due to aspartame? Who can tell? Even if it was, does it matter to most of the population? Rarely, people have an adverse reaction to aspirin, but it is so rare that aspirin is readily available without prescription; nobody suggests that it should be banned. It may be that some individuals react to a food item in an unusual and extreme way, but usually most of us do not. There is little evidence that most children react to a drink containing aspartame in a predictable way.

The possibility that a lifetime of consuming aspartame may have a cumulative impact is another matter, one that has hardly been considered. A long-term impact is a possibility that should not be ignored, although it is unclear how the intake of aspartame could be monitored over a period of years.

Some of the concern about aspartame reflects its chemical

structure. It consists of two amino acids, phenylalanine and aspartate. Amino acids are the basic units from which protein is built. Does the use of the sweetener increase the levels of phenylalanine in the brain to the extent that they are harmful?

When we are born, the medical profession routinely screens us for a genetic disorder, phenylketonuria (PKU). Those with the disorder lack the ability to metabolize phenylalanine in the usual manner, and the abnormal chemicals that result cause brain damage and severe mental retardation. Fortunately, the disorder can be identified at birth, and if a diet low in phenylalanine is provided, then development is relatively normal. The low-phenylalanine diet is usually fed until brain development has taken place. Those with PKU but no longer on a restricted diet have become concerned about taking aspartame. Will aspartame increase the levels of phenylalanine in the brain and cause problems? For those on a phenylalanine-restricted diet aspartame will be a major source of the amino acid. To alert interested individuals, food labels now contain warnings such as 'Phenylketonurics: Contains Phenylalanine'.

Another group that are advised to avoid aspartame are those with a history of depression. Ralph Walton, a psychiatrist working in Ohio, wondered if aspartame might influence those aspects of the brain chemistry that are associated with depression. Phenylalanine is converted into dopamine and noradrenaline, two of the chemicals that send messages between brain cells. He had observed in his clinical practice that depressed patients appeared to respond adversely to drinks containing aspartame. He gave patients with a history of major depression either aspartame or a placebo for seven days. The response was so marked that the ethical committee that was overseeing the study insisted that it was stopped before it was due to finish.[29] Three out of eight depressed patients used the term 'poisoned' to describe how they felt. Two developed serious eye problems, which led to the study being ended. Those who were not depressed did not report any effect of taking aspartame. Although this is the only study that has looked at depressed patients, as a precaution it is sensible to discourage those with this disorder from taking aspartame.

## *Sugar – nice but naughty?*

This chapter has looked at three related questions. Do some individuals react adversely to sugar? Are low levels of blood glucose a cause for concern? Does a high-sugar diet induce wide swings in the level of blood glucose? It is apparent that the question 'Is sugar bad for you psychologically?' is posed in too simple a manner. It can be both beneficial and harmful, depending on the rest of the diet, which aspect of behaviour is being examined and how you, as an individual, respond.

For some of us, our physiology is such that we can have problems caused by either food intolerance or the development of low blood glucose. There is no doubt that in susceptible individuals sugar in the diet can produce an adverse effect. The frequency with which such responses occur should be placed in context; they are uncommon. A study of the foods to which hyperactive children respond found sixteen other foods to which children responded more often than sugar (see Table 6.3). Only 16 per cent of children responded to sugar, whereas 64 per cent responded to cow's milk, 59 per cent to chocolate and 49 per cent to grapes and wheat.[30] There was less reason to single out sugar as a problem than many other foods.

Common sense would seem to suggest that sugar should lead to particularly large increases in blood glucose, yet the picture is less clear than might be expected. For many years the advice to those suffering with food-induced hypoglycaemia was to eat complex rather than simple carbohydrates. Complex carbohydrates include pasta, potatoes, rice and grain products. More recently, it has become apparent that there are large differences in the reaction to complex carbohydrates.[31] Each has a different action on blood glucose. Cooked potato causes blood glucose levels to increase more than cooked rice does. Potatoes cause just as large a release of insulin as pure sugar, although it is about thirty minutes slower. The insulin response to bread is similar to its response to potatoes and sugar. In contrast, rice and corn cause a smaller reaction. There are marked individual differences in the reactions to foods. In reactive individuals complex carbohydrates can have a similar influence on blood glucose as sugar will have in a less reactive person.

A glucose drink can have short-term benefits, for example with the forge workers (Figure 7.4) and in the driving simulator (Figure 7.5). It is a cliché that there is no such thing as a bad food, only a bad diet. Whether the amount of food eaten is a problem depends on not only how much is eaten but also what else is, or is not, consumed.

The comment that sugar provides empty calories has been made frequently. The implication is that if too many calories come in the form of sugar, then the diet might be deficient in vitamins and minerals. In fact, dietary surveys have tended to find that in adults a high sugar intake is not associated with a particularly low intake of micronutrients. The reason is that most people eating a large amount of sugar also eat large amounts of other foods, which contain micronutrients. The levels of minerals and vitamins in the body are more closely related to total energy intake than to sugar intake. A particular problem occurs if people consume a low-calorie diet that obtains a high proportion of those calories in the form of sugar.[32] This combines two aspects of diet that are associated with a low micronutrient intake: a low-calorie and a high-sugar diet. These conclusions are based on studies of the diet of adults. It is obvious that children might have particular problems, although the topic has been little explored.

If a low-calorie, high-sugar diet is a potential problem, then some children must be at risk. When the parents of 6-year-old children were asked, 93 per cent said that their children always or frequently ate snacks or sweets in place of meals. Fifteen per cent of children had a poor diet and regularly picked at their meals.[33] Does this imply that some children combine a low-calorie input (low appetite) and high-sugar diet? If so, then they are at a high risk of consuming only marginal amounts of vitamins and minerals. Clearly, this is a possibility that should be seriously considered.

The impact of vitamin–mineral supplementation on performance on intelligence tests was discussed in Chapter 4. Richard Cook in Swansea, Wales, found that the intelligence scores of 6-year-old children increased by over seven points after taking vitamin–mineral supplements for two months, whereas in those taking a placebo the scores fell 1.7 points.[34] Sugar intake was estimated by asking the frequency with which particular foods were eaten. The more sugar in the diet, the greater was the response to vitamin–mineral supplements. This finding needs to be interpreted cautiously. Did those children with a high sugar intake have a low vitamin intake? We do not know. It is an obvious suggestion, but the measure of sugar consumption was crude and there was no measure of vitamin intake. Without a series of similar studies it is difficult to establish the extent of the relationship.

Western nations have a love–hate relationship with sugar. It is an innately attractive substance; when given a choice a newborn child will choose a sweet taste rather than an alternative. Sugars in berries, fruit and honey have always formed part of the human diet. With increasing affluence, we have available more sweet-tasting food than we can eat. There have been claims, always contested, that sugar intake predisposes people to a variety of diseases: dental caries, diabetes mellitus, cardiovascular disease, obesity and behavioural problems.[35] However, any general statements about sugar have always proved too simple; this is true of behavioural as well as physical complaints.

# CHAPTER 8

# Diet and Violence

Soccer hooliganism and teenage delinquency could be curbed by giving young people healthier food, two nutritionists claimed ... 'You cannot hope for good behaviour on a junk food diet, whatever social improvements are made. It is affecting behaviour patterns, especially in young males. Analysis of the diet of football hooligans would show a huge amount of nutritional deficiencies.'[1]

What do you make of such a claim? It is likely to be criticized from every perspective. Nutritionists will point to dietary surveys to demonstrate that widespread deficiencies do not exist (but see Chapter 2 to understand the faith that can be placed in such surveys). Sociologists will stress the predominant importance of a subculture in which football violence is the means of gaining social status. Even many people who are predisposed to believe that diet may influence behaviour will wish to distance themselves from such remarks. Few would believe that giving football supporters vitamin tablets, or in other ways changing their diets, would have anything other than a minor impact on their behaviour.

The idea that changing the diet of violent criminals will decrease their aggressive behaviour owes much to two Americans. Barbara Reed, a senior probation officer in Ohio, claimed remarkable success when she tried to rehabilitate young offenders by putting them on a low-sugar, no junk-food diet. In 1977 she testified before the US Select Committee on Nutrition and Human Needs. The diet she used was low in refined sugar and flour, food additives, coffee and coffee substitutes, soft drinks, grapes, prunes, dates, raisins, figs, all refined starch foods, caffeine and alcoholic drinks.

She told the Senate Committee that in over 250 cases 'we have not had one single person back in court who has stayed on the diet'.[2]

The following year Alexander Schauss, who was also a probation officer, published his book *Diet, Crime and Delinquency*.[3] In this bestseller he described how a low-sugar diet decreased violent behaviour.

Although the publicity was sufficient to encourage several American probation departments to adopt a dietary approach, more typically it was greeted with scepticism. There was little that could be considered hard evidence. Certainly, if the approach worked, it was unclear why it worked: with so many changes to the diet it was impossible to know what was happening. Was it the removal of caffeine, alcohol, additives, sugar or something else that was important? Was it the foods that were removed, or the new foods that were introduced, that were critical? Without comparison groups, can it be certain that there was more than a placebo response?

Everything we know about human behaviour stresses the vast importance of social and cultural factors in its determination. Scientists would need powerful evidence before concluding that diet played the major role. Having said this, a poor diet may play at least a part in predisposing some of us towards irritability. In a few of us an inability of our body to deal adequately with some food items can dramatically induce aggressive behaviour. The three major means by which diet may induce an aggressive tendency have all been introduced: food intolerance, low blood glucose, and vitamin and mineral deficiencies.

## Food intolerance

In 1978 the Mayor of San Francisco, George Moscone, was killed by another politician, Dan White. White's lawyer pleaded diminished responsibility, on the grounds that his client's brain function had been diminished by a junk-food diet. The jury agreed and White was convicted of manslaughter rather than murder. The verdict was so unexpected that the state passed a law banning the 'bad diet' defence.

Irrespective of whether you think that your decision to eat a particular diet should make you legally less responsible for your own behaviour, there is little doubt that in a minority of people food intolerance can induce antisocial behaviour. That food intolerance may cause violent behaviour can be illustrated by the case of Joanna, described in Chapter 5, who displayed aggression to both her children and herself. The careful use of a double-blind approach means that, in her case, we can be certain that food intolerance caused her aggressive behaviour. Although day-to-day clinical observation lacks the certainty of the experimental approach, it supports the suggestion that we should expect food-induced aggressive behaviour elsewhere in the population. William Crook, a paediatrician in Tennessee, reported the comments of parents whose children he had treated by eliminating certain items of food from their diet:

Charlie was expelled from nursery school at eighteen months for aggressive behavior. His worst food trouble-makers were red dye, peanuts, wheat, sugar and milk. We continue to control his diet and peanut is the main food that still gives him trouble. Today, at four and a half, Charlie continues to be an extraordinary contrast to what he was two and a half years ago. His mental capacities are, to say the least, astounding. He sleeps well, rarely awakens in the night; also he hasn't had an infection requiring antibiotics in months. Instead of being the most trouble of four children, he's by far now the least.

. . .

Joe has been on a limited diet for five years. He can eat a small amount of some of the offending foods, but simply cannot handle in any amount milk, red dye or potatoes. His whole behavior pattern changes drastically when he slips and eats these foods. Milk causes him to exhibit hostile behavior and to wet the bed everytime he drinks even one ounce. It's as obvious as if he wore a sign saying 'I drank milk.' And red colors, citrus and potatoes make him hyperactive and irritable. The elimination diet has literally been a life-saver for Joe and our family.[4]

The owner of a Yorkshire residential home for individuals with learning disabilities writes:

The majority of our residents are initially heavily medicated to control aggressive/disruptive behaviours. Many have inflicted horrific self injuries and have been diagnosed as schizophrenic or autistic. Their crimes range from murder, arson, joy riding and sexual offences to petty theft. Their assessed mental ages range from between six to twelve years.

We first became aware that diet can influence behaviour when a twenty-three-year-old lady who, having spent her formative years in local authority care and three years in a psychiatric hospital, was referred to us. Having been controlled by massive doses of anti-psychotic drugs, diagnosed as schizophrenic, low mentality and exhibiting behavioural problems (aggression and self mutilation), it transpired that she could not tolerate many foods and her behaviour was influenced by her diet. Her diet was changed and she is now virtually free from all medication, has been living a relatively independent life in the community and has two lovely children.

A controlled diet is obviously not the only answer to anti-social behaviour, but we have found it does play a major part, especially when trying to reduce often unnecessarily prescribed medication.[5]

This home could function only with the assistance of the local general practitioner, who commented:

I have seen three patients who were previously diagnosed as having epilepsy causing mood disorders leading to anti-social behaviour. In each case we have been able to slowly reduce anti-epileptic and other major sedating medication with no adverse epileptic nor behavioural effects.[6]

It seems reasonable to assume that some cases of extreme violence reflect food intolerance. A court in Belfast was prepared to take food intolerance into account when a young man pleaded guilty to assault. He was given a conditional discharge when it was accepted that eating potatoes had altered his personality. It is, however, equally certain that the majority of those rioting at a football match are not reacting to food intolerance. It would be particularly interesting to study people in prison who have a history of violent crime. It would not be surprising if some, but not all, of these violent prisoners were found to have food intolerance.

## *Low blood sugar*

Perhaps the most common mechanism that is suggested to be associated with violence is hypoglycaemia – that is, low blood glucose. A
basic argument offered by Alexander Schauss was that a diet containing large amounts of refined sugar would be associated with a tendency to develop low levels of blood glucose, to the extent that the
functioning of the brain is disrupted. Although Chapter 7 argued
that hypoglycaemia occurs rarely in response to a normal diet, it
may be that a greater fall in blood glucose is more likely to occur in
those with a history of violence.

### Qolla Indians

The Qolla Indians, who live at a high altitude in Peru, are known
for their high murder rate and family feuds. Among anthropologists
their claim to fame is that:

these Andean highlanders are portrayed as perhaps the meanest and most
unlikeable people on earth;[7]
. . .

[they are] the classic example of a people with an extreme modal personality
dominated by excesses of hostility and aggressiveness;[8]
. . .

[they] tend to swagger, especially when inebriated, and at such times they
frequently indulge in monologues describing their own ferocity while laugh-
ing at the puniness of their enemies . . . they shout 'You are nothing but a
dog, an ass, excrement.'[9]

Most attempts by anthropologists to explain the behaviour of
the Qolla have relied on cultural explanations. Their behaviour was
said to reflect years of domination by the Incas and the Spanish;
alternatively, emphasis was placed on the harshness of their environment, particularly the high altitude and lack of food. Neither are
very convincing explanations. It is easy to point to people in other
parts of the world who have a history of being dominated, or who
live at a similar altitude, without being extremely aggressive.

A markedly different explanation was offered by Ralph Bolton, an American anthropologist.[10] He noted that many acts of violence appeared to be irrational, even to the Qolla, as they were stimulated by the most minor of events. A violent response was not culturally approved. Rather, some of the Qolla were viewed as extremely irritable and were thought to respond inappropriately to minor problems. Ralph Bolton wondered if the aggression of the Qolla was a reaction to food. He noticed a strong craving for sugar and that many people had an almost insatiable hunger. He considered the possibility that their aggressiveness reflected a tendency to develop low levels of blood glucose.

Bolton gave male Qolla a Glucose Tolerance Test (see Chapter 7). After fasting overnight, the men drank 50 grams of glucose, and the initial rise and subsequent fall in blood glucose was monitored for four hours. The extent to which blood glucose levels fell below the initial values was the measure taken. Three Qolla rated members of their group for their degree of aggressiveness. Those who were ranked as most aggressive had a tendency for their blood glucose to fall farther in a Glucose Tolerance Test.

The Qolla were also asked to complete sentences such as: 'A family . . .'. Such open-ended questions allow psychologists to gain some insight into the way that people think. There is a large range of possible answers, which were analysed for aggressive content. Those who developed low blood glucose levels proved more likely to complete sentences with an aggressive content, for example, 'A family needs to fight in order to survive.' Thus those with a tendency to develop low blood glucose levels not only acted aggressively, but they also thought aggressive thoughts.

### Violent criminals

Matti Virkkunen, a psychiatrist who works in Helsinki, has repeatedly found a characteristic pattern of blood glucose changes in people who have committed a range of violent crimes.[11] Offenders who had committed one or more severe violent assaults have been examined in prison. In a Glucose Tolerance Test their blood glucose levels rose to abnormally high levels and later fell to particularly low values, from which they were slow to recover. Similarly, a tendency to develop low levels of blood glucose has been found in those with antisocial personalities. These observations have been followed up by measuring insulin secretion. Insulin is the hormone that, when released from the pancreas, stimulates the removal of glucose from the bloodstream. It seems that some violent offenders react to increases in blood glucose by releasing high levels of insulin, which, in turn, causes the level of blood glucose to fall rapidly.[12]

There is an interesting association between violence, the drinking of alcohol and a tendency for low blood glucose levels to develop. Violent criminals who had committed crimes following the taking of alcohol also tended to have low blood glucose values during a glucose test. Alcohol facilitates the ability of glucose to stimulate the secretion of insulin. Thus the combination of alcohol and rising blood glucose levels is associated with a particularly large release of insulin, which results in rapidly falling blood glucose values. It may be relevant that people with an antisocial personality are particularly likely to commit violent crimes while under the influence of alcohol – a situation when blood glucose levels fall rapidly.[13]

### Blood glucose aggression and the normal population

Both the Qolla Indians and the Finnish violent offenders are atypical in that they displayed extreme violence. Is the association between falling blood glucose and aggression an abnormal response of a few very violent individuals, or is there a similar tendency throughout the population?

Normal male members of British society were presented with a series of cartoons that depicted frustrating situations, such as being splashed by a passing car. In this example they were asked what the person who was splashed by the car was likely to have said. It is assumed that such projective tests allow feelings to be expressed in an indirect manner when socially unacceptable comments may otherwise be inhibited. The extent to which the responses were aggressive was assessed. The subjects were also asked to say to what extent they approved of aggressive acts. A series of situations was presented and the extent to which it was thought justified to use different types of aggression – killing, hitting, shouting – or gentle persuasion was recorded. The men whose levels of blood glucose fell rapidly in a Glucose Tolerance Test were more likely to include aggressive comments when faced with the frustrating cartoons; they were more likely to think that aggressive acts were justified. It seems that throughout the population people whose blood glucose levels fall rapidly have a tendency to think aggressive thoughts and to approve of aggressive acts.[14]

## Does low blood glucose cause aggression?

Attempts to relate the intake of sugar, hypoglycaemia and violent behaviour attract several types of criticism. Firstly, in case of the Qolla Indians, Finnish prisoners and British males all we have is a correlation. As always, we cannot assume that diet-induced changes in blood glucose levels necessarily cause aggressive behaviour. A distinct possibility is that a third factor, maybe a hormone or a brain chemical, influences both aggression and blood glucose. One way of establishing that blood glucose does predispose towards aggression is to alter blood glucose levels while monitoring the level of aggression. This approach is easy to recommend, but in practice not easy to achieve. In adults both cultural and legal inhibitions make the expression of overt physical aggression unlikely. Aggression tends to come as an occasional explosive event, and it is therefore difficult to monitor continuous changes over short periods of time. For these reasons, one of the few studies of this question was carried out using children, whose behaviour is more spontaneous and whose aggression tends to be less restrained.[15]

Normal 6- to 7-year-olds without any history of behavioural problems were subjected to a frustrating situation and their reactions monitored. They played with a television computer game in which an electronic representation of a ball moved across the screen. The task was to turn a knob that placed an electronic bat in the way of the ball. The difficulty of the task could be altered by adjusting the speed of the ball, the size of the bat and the angle at which the ball left the wall. The conditions were chosen to be the most difficult. In fact, without extensive practice the game was next to impossible for an adult; a child was bound to fail. The question was how did the children react to failure?

Their behaviour was observed. Did they show signs of frustration; did they handle the controls roughly, kick their feet, were they restless, did they sigh or express annoyance? Towards the end of a school day the children received a drink containing glucose or a placebo. When faced with the impossible video game, those who received the glucose drink were markedly less likely to display signs of frustration and irritability. Although this study demonstrated what parents have known for generations, that hungry children are irritable, it had been shown for the first time that experimentally increasing blood glucose levels decreased irritability. It is important that the observation was made in normal children. It appeared that blood glucose levels were important not only in a few extremely violent individuals.

Later, the same impossible computer game was given to young adults without any history of antisocial behaviour, and their reaction to the frustration was monitored.[16] If they grimaced, hit the equipment, swore, made negative comments or sighed, this was noted. There was relatively little evidence of negative behaviour; it is not socially accepted to act in this manner. As this had been expected, at a predetermined stage an attractive female experimenter said to the male subjects, 'Most people are better by now'. The intention was that this remark would irritate the subjects. It did. As you see in Figure 8.1, the comment greatly increased the irritable behaviour that was observed, but less so if the subject had had a drink containing glucose. Thus in a second double-blind study, consuming a glucose drink decreased irritability. Again, the response occurred in normal members of the population without a history of violence, and it occurred when blood glucose levels had not fallen to the low levels needed to diagnose clinical hypoglycaemia.

The second criticism directed towards people who suggest that low blood glucose levels predispose to aggression is that hypoglycaemia occurs rarely. There is little doubt that few of the Qolla Indians, Finnish offenders and British males satisfy the clinical criteria that would allow a diagnosis of reactive hypoglycaemia. Blood glucose simply did not fall to levels where, in a clinical sense,

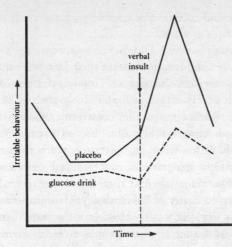

*Figure 8.1* **Blood glucose level and irritable behaviour**
Irritable behaviour was monitored while failing at an impossible
computer game following either a placebo or glucose drink. Note
that when the experimenter commented adversely about their
performance, the incidence of negative behaviours increased less in
those who had had a glucose drink.
*Source:* Benton and Owens, *Journal of Psychosomatic Research*, 37, 1993,
723–35.

it can be described as hypoglycaemic. It is true that in normal
individuals, fed in a usual manner, a hypoglycaemic response is uncommon. It has, however, become increasingly clear that blood
glucose levels higher than those that can be described as hypoglycaemic may limit cognitive functioning (see Chapter 7).

Moderate falls in blood glucose may cause irritability. Whether
it leads to aggressive behaviour depends on provocation, social skills
and other aspects of the situation. It should be realized that these
studies of blood glucose levels demonstrate marked individual differences in the response to diet. They tell us not about a general reaction
to diet, but emphasize that we all react to our diet in different ways.
Some of us have a tendency to develop low blood glucose levels and
become irritable; for others this is less of a problem.

## *Vitamin and mineral intake*

Steven Schoenthaler is a Californian criminologist and the first person to obtain systematic data relating the intake of sugar to violent behaviour. Much of his early work was stimulated by the suggestion of Alexander Schauss that a diet containing substantial amounts of highly refined sugar would induce hypoglycaemia. As we will see, the emphasis of his work has changed over the years from sugar to the possibility that problems are caused by a low intake of vitamins and minerals.

The approach taken in many of his studies was similar. In a juvenile detention facility the diet was changed with the stated aim of decreasing the intake of sugar. Typical changes included giving honey rather than sugar; fruit, cheese or nuts rather than high-sugar desserts; fruit juice rather than soft drinks; unsweetened cereals instead of presweetened cereals.

All prisons in the United States are required to record every antisocial act in an incident report book. The items recorded vary from minor events, such as verbal abuse or insubordination, to more serious ones, such as vandalism, theft and violent assaults. The disciplinary records of institutions before and after changing the diet were compared. On the basis of these studies it is claimed that the incidence of antisocial behaviour declined between 21 and 54 per cent.

For example, in a juvenile detention centre in Virginia the number of disciplinary incidents almost halved in the year following a change in diet.[17] Unfortunately, diet was not the only change that occurred. The proportion of females increased, and the age and the proportion of white and non-white prisoners altered in directions that could be expected to decrease the number of reported incidents. In many institutions staff have discretion as to whether they report an incident. It is very likely that having been given the expectation that misbehaviour would decrease, the way that behaviour was viewed would change. The other studies in this series suffer from similar problems. The results are, however, sufficiently consistent for a more experimental study to be of interest.

If you believe that the change in diet was causing the decrease in antisocial behaviour, and many people did not, it is unclear why it was happening. There are three possible mechanisms.

1 Eating foods containing high levels of refined sugar might cause reactive hypoglycaemia. The resulting low blood glucose levels would be expected to impair brain functioning.

2 Foods with high levels of sugar tend to have more than their share of colourings, artificial flavours and preservatives. These additives may have induced an allergic or other type of adverse reaction.

3 As sugar is highly refined and contains few vitamins and minerals, a high-sugar diet may provide inadequate levels of micronutrients. In this way the brain's chemistry is impaired.

The time-scale of the changes pointed towards the third of these explanations. The improvement in behaviour occurred gradually over a period of about eighteen weeks, after which it remained constant.[18] If hypoglycaemia or food intolerance caused the antisocial behaviour, the removal of the offending food items from the diet would produce a rapid improvement in behaviour. If there was a minor deficiency of vitamins and minerals, then an improved diet would be expected to gradually replace the micronutrients over a period of weeks.

Steven Schoenthaler next studied young offenders, guilty of serious crimes, in two penal institutions in California and Florida.[19] He recorded everything they chose to eat for seven days and calculated the intake of a range of nutrients. It is commonly suggested that if a person consumes less than 70 per cent of the RDA, then this is a cause for concern. Schoenthaler distinguished those individuals whose diet offered less than 70 per cent of the RDA in the case of at least five nutrients (poorly nourished group) from those with a better diet. The official incident records were examined for the previous year and those who had committed offences were distinguished from those who had not. Figure 8.2 shows that those with the poorer diet were significantly more likely to have committed serious offences. As these offences had been recorded in the previous year, there was no way that the behaviour of either the staff or

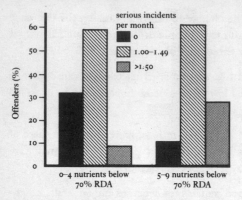

*Figure 8.2* **Micronutrients in the diet and antisocial behaviour**
Diet was recorded for seven days and the number of micronutrients
consumed at levels lower than 70 per cent of the RDA were calculated.
Individuals with a poorer diet committed more antisocial acts.
*Source:* Schoenthaler, *International Journal of Biosocial Research*, 5, 1983,
99–106.

the inmates could have been influenced by taking part in an experiment; that is, there was no possibility that the difference in behaviour
was a placebo response.

These findings were, however, simply a correlation; better diet
and better behaviour were associated. Did a better diet cause better
behaviour or did those with better behaviour choose a better diet?
Were both better behaviour and the choice of a better diet simply a
reflection of a better upbringing? A double-blind study was required.

A multi-vitamin and mineral supplement was given for three
months to all offenders, irrespective of the quality of their diet. It
was argued that those with a poor diet would respond, as they had
less than optimal stores of micronutrients. The behaviour of those
who ate a better diet would not be expected to improve because the
diet already supplied all the vitamins and minerals that were needed.
Mood and behaviour were compared for the three months before
and after taking the supplements. It was found that if the subjects
had a poor diet, taking a vitamin–mineral supplement improved
their mood, they became less angry (Figure 8.3). If the subjects' diet

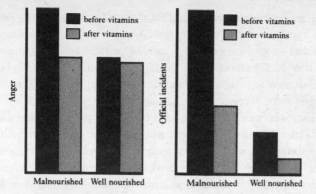

*Figure 8.3* **Vitamin–mineral supplementation and antisocial behaviour**

The behaviour of juvenile delinquents in detention centres was compared three months before and three months after taking vitamin–mineral supplements. Those whose diet supplied vitamins at the RDA were distinguished from those whose diet provided less than 70 per cent of the RDA. Incidents of misbehaviour and self-reported anger decreased in those who had a poor diet and took supplements.

*Source:* Data from Schoenthaler, in Essman, *Nutrients and Brain Function.*

was good to begin with, taking a supplement was without effect. Similarly, if the subjects ate a poor diet, taking the supplement decreased misbehaviour, but if their diet was good, the extra vitamins and minerals were without effect.[20] This study was said to be double-blind in that neither the staff nor the offenders were aware whose diet offered an intake of nutrients less than 70 per cent of the RDA.

Scientists are trained to be small-minded; rightly, they should point out even the most improbable of potential problems. It is possible that when the vitamin tablets were introduced, the attention of the staff became focused on what the offenders were eating. It may have been possible to distinguish those who obviously consumed a nutritionally inadequate diet from those who ate a much better diet. If this occurred, then the study would no longer have been double-blind and there would be grounds to doubt the results.

Again, all we have is a correlation. Did those who chose to eat a poor diet also choose to behave in antisocial ways? A good experiment requires that people are randomly placed in the various treatment groups; this had not occurred. Such arguments may seem far-fetched, but no matter now improbable they sound, it can be claimed that there is a doubt concerning the findings.

What was needed was a double-blind placebo-controlled study. Randomly, some offenders needed to be given a vitamin-mineral supplement while others took a placebo. Only then could scientists be sure that the results were valid. Stephen Schoenthaler gave either a vitamin-mineral supplement or placebo under double-blind conditions to sixty-four juveniles in a treatment facility. The taking of a vitamin-mineral supplement was associated with significantly less violent behaviour, less non-violent antisocial behaviour and fewer assaults on staff. A good micronutrient profile, either originally or following supplementation, was a better indicator of good behaviour than whether the active tablet or a placebo had been taken.

The data has been collected, but not yet published, in the first large-scale double-blind placebo-controlled study of the vitamin-mineral supplementation of incarcerated adults.[21] In this study of 406 subjects the taking of the supplement was associated with a significant decrease in the incidence of rule breaking. The publication of this study is awaited with great anticipation. Researchers will wish to examine the report in detail but the work was funded by the State of California and the design and implementation was overseen by a committee of well qualified, sceptical academics and professionals. Their role was to ensure that the experiment met the highest possible standards.

## What is decreasing violence?

Steven Schoenthaler's research on diet and violence has, over many years, examined the hypothesis that the level of sugar in the diet is important. No convincing evidence that this is the case has been collected. The dietary changes that were introduced were extensive.

It follows that the intake of a wide range of nutrients changed. Therefore it was not reasonable to conclude that any particular nutrient was more important than any other. As the studies have become progressively better designed it has become apparent that a shortage of vitamins and minerals in the diet seems to be important. And as the research has edged towards the ideal of double-blind placebo studies we can be more certain of this conclusion.

To date Steven Schoenthaler is the only person who has begun to look at the topic of vitamin–mineral intake and antisocial behaviour. As always happens when you advocate a scientifically unfashionable idea, he has attracted a great deal of personal criticism. It is to be hoped that others will look at the topic. Only when a number of independent researchers report similar results will the underlying ideas become widely accepted.

## Diet – a suitable means of treatment?

Terry, a thin, unhealthy-looking 17-year-old, slouched into a North of England court. Having a long history of convictions for burglaries, he had expected to be remanded in custody until his trial for sixty other similar offences. Instead, at the request of a probation officer, he was given bail and given into the charge of South Cumbrian Alternative Sentencing Option (SCASO), a charity in Barrow in Furness that tries to keep youngsters out of custody. Three weeks later Terry was back in court and the magistrate commented that he could hardly believe that this was the same person. He appeared confident and his face had some colour.

SCASO, under its director Bernard Gesch, believes that food and environmental toxins stimulate a great deal of antisocial behaviour. Supported by a small grant from the local authority, the organization has found it surprisingly easy to persuade magistrates to allow it to explore the impact of changing diet on delinquent behaviour. Terry had started a crash course of vitamins and minerals, and intolerance to various foods had been established. Unlike the four previous occasions when he had appeared in court, he left without a prison sentence; he went back to live with his parents. With a new diet, he grew taller and put on a stone in weight in six months. His behaviour and self-confidence improved, he started a job and no longer craved sweets or wanted to sniff glue.

Terry is only one of many successes claimed by SCASO, although when his parents separated, he went back to his old diet of junk food and to his old criminal ways. Bernard Gesch commented about changing the eating habits of delinquents:

We start slowly. If they eat burgers we suggest they substitute a proper piece of meat and that they change from white to brown bread. We suggest sugar-free baked beans are better than chips and that vegetables from the green grocers are better than from tins. Some eat a catastrophic amount of sugar. As they start to get better, sometimes for the first time in years, they become more and more responsive. Families are also positive. They tend to feel that they have been blamed for the way they brought up their child. If they are on income support they find it hard to afford a healthy diet.

One girl who was referred to us was about to be sent to secure accommodation costing six hundred pounds a week. We worked out that to change her diet and give her supplements cost four pounds a day.

I have worked with juvenile offenders for years and have yet to see anything which has such a sledge-hammer on a plate-glass window effect as this.[22]

What are we to make of such cases? Although the approach of SCASO has attracted the support of some magistrates, many of the local social workers and probation officers are resistant to the idea that diet plays such an important role. Scientists looking for hard evidence will see case studies such as these as uninterpretable.

It is unreasonable to criticize such attempts to help people with serious problems as unscientific. A treatment centre is not trying to run a scientific study. Rather, ideas based on previous scientific work are being used to help others. Having said this, case studies are indeed difficult to interpret. There is a considerable element of judgement and good fortune in coming to a correct diagnosis, and hence the appropriate treatment.

Was the behavioural improvement of the youngsters helped by SCASO due only to diet? It is impossible to be sure. Being sent to a centre that specializes in keeping youngsters out of gaol may, for the first time in years, allow the offender to interact with dedicated adults who are interested in their well-being. It is impossible to exclude the possibility that changes in the social and psychological environment may have helped to change behaviour. It would be strange if they did not. Without a double-blind procedure it is impossible to exclude the possibility that any improvement is more than a placebo response.

On the other hand, there can be little doubt that food intolerance can induce antisocial behaviour; double-blind trials have demonstrated that this is the case. Thus it is reasonable to expect that at least some children with a history of violent and antisocial behaviour will have a problem with food intolerance. It is, however, unclear how often violence is a reflection of food intolerance. The evidence that a poor micronutrient status may predispose people to violent behaviour remains controversial, although the evidence in favour of the proposition is growing. Accepting the general message that aspects of the diet influence behaviour, correctional facilities in several American states have modified diets, expecting improvements in behaviour. The enthusiastic way in which many public agencies have taken up the idea that diet influences criminal behaviour has led to professional concern. The California Council Against Health Fraud issued a statement, later endorsed by the American Dietetic Association:

Valid evidence is lacking to support the claim that diet is an important determinant in the development of violence and criminal behavior.
. . .
Valid evidence is lacking to support the hypothesis that reactive hypoglycemia is a common cause for violent behavior.
. . .
Those who profess that there is a link between diet and criminal behavior often point to foods that are the popular whipping boys, such as processed foods containing refined sugar and white flour . . . however, many other foods . . . for example, both milk and oranges have been singled out as 'problem' foods by some who promote the unfounded belief that brain 'allergies' are a major cause of violence and criminal behavior.
. . .
Evidence used to support such beliefs may sound dramatic, but it is largely

subjective evidence presented by believers. This evidence consists primarily of anecdotal case reports, and reports of studies that have not been conducted under carefully controlled conditions.[23]

Much of the warning of the group concerned with health fraud can be justified if you emphasize the qualifications 'important determinant', 'common cause', 'major cause'. Does diet influence aggression rarely or is it a common problem? There is no way of answering this key question. The probability is that for most young offenders diet is neither the cause of nor the means of solving their problems. In some it may be a contributory factor. For a minority, diet may be driving their antisocial behaviour; the size of that minority is anybody's guess.

It is totally unreasonable to see diet as 'the' cause of aggressive behaviour. It is unreasonable to view aggression as a switch that diet turns on or off. At the most, diet creates a predisposition. Whether that predisposition ends up as a violent act depends on a range of other factors. Although the blood glucose levels of the most aggressive Qolla Indians tended to fall more rapidly than those who were less aggressive, there was no simple relationship. A few of the most aggressive Qolla had normal blood glucose reactions. A few of the

*Figure 8.4* **Advice for the irritable**

---

1 If you think that your irritable nature reflects your diet, then think again. Are you sure that there is nothing else about the demands of your life that explains the way you are?

2 If your feelings of irritability correspond with particular times of day, then you might consider a dietary explanation. If you regularly feel low in the late afternoon, or in the late morning if you go without breakfast, then a change in diet may help.

3 The solution is straightforward. Do not miss meals. Instead of three meals, consider eating a little and often, although be sure not to increase your calorie intake. Ensure that you consume a varied diet that contains unrefined carbohydrates and a range of fruit and vegetables.

---

least aggressive Qolla displayed very large falls in blood glucose. Although violent criminals were more likely to have blood glucose levels that fell rapidly, there are normal members of society, without a history of violent crime, who are similar in this respect. The day has not yet come when all those entering a football ground should be offered a vitamin pill.

# CHAPTER 9

# Too Little or Too Much of a Good Thing?

The sale of vitamin supplements is a multi-million-pound industry. Chains of shops survive by selling nothing other than vitamin supplements and related products. It has been estimated that each day 50 to 60 million Americans swallow vitamin and mineral supplements. There are three reasons why you might believe that taking extra vitamins will do you some good:

1 Your diet supplies vitamins in insufficient amounts.

2 You have a genetically determined need for more than the average intake.

3 Very large amounts of vitamins act in a similar manner to drugs, in which case the vitamin is taken not as a food supplement but for its pharmaceutical properties.

There are few human complaints that have not been said to respond to the taking of one vitamin or another. In the present chapter only psychological complaints and only some of the vitamins that have attracted particular attention are considered.

## Megavitamins

It is well established that vitamins and minerals are an important part of the diet and that a deficiency can have both physical and psychological consequences. If a small deficiency can have adverse psychological consequences, is it possible that a greater than normal supply can offer additional benefits?

Megavitamin therapy got a great boost in 1968 when Linus Pauling, who had received the Nobel prize for chemistry, proposed that large concentrations of vitamins can benefit the body. He suggested that the benefits may be physical, for example you are less likely to suffer with the common cold if you take vitamin C, or they may be psychological, as mental imbalances develop as a result of nutritional deficiencies. Pauling defined orthomolecular psychiatry as the 'treatment of mental disease by the provision of the optimum molecular environment for the mind'.[1] Although often thought of as being synonymous with the use of vitamins in large doses, in particular cases it may also involve a decreased intake.

Megavitamin therapy has been defined as treatment with doses of vitamins that exceed ten times the RDA; in fact, doses that are hundreds or even thousands of times the RDA are used. In Pauling's view some forms of mental illness reflect a vitamin deficiency that results from a diet that in many of the population would be adequate. We differ in the extent to which our basic biology is able to ensure that critical nutrients reach those areas of the brain where they are needed. Controversially, Pauling proposed that while the rest of the body had adequate amounts of a vitamin, the brain might be deficient. For example, while you might not have the bodily symptoms of the deficiency disease pellagra, you might have the symptoms associated with a low supply of niacin to the brain.

A related idea is that there is considerable biological individuality. In the same way that no two snowflakes are identical, no two bodies are the same. The need for vitamins can differ by several hundred per cent.[2]

It has been claimed that high levels of vitamins may benefit a range of behavioural problems: schizophrenia, mental retardation, hyperactivity and autism. The nature of the evidence on which such claims are based has set apart those who take the orthomolecular approach. Double-blind trials are viewed as unethical, as half the patients are denied a 'valuable treatment' when they are offered a placebo. Nutritional needs are seen as individual, therefore it makes little sense to give the same supplements to a large group. Instead, case studies are quoted, often with apparently dramatic improvements. For people taking the more traditional scientific approach, the failure of double-blind studies to support most of the claims is seen as damning.

The use of a small dose of vitamins to make good a possible dietary shortfall can be termed a food supplement. This needs to be distinguished from the use of megavitamins, intakes vastly in excess of the recommended level. To ensure that these two approaches are distinguished, when any study is mentioned the dose of vitamin used will be reported in terms of the British RDAs.

## Thiamine

Vitamin $B_1$, or thiamine, is widely distributed in foods but is easily destroyed by boiling. As the body has only small stores of thiamine there is a risk of deficiency if the level of intake is reduced for only a few weeks. Thiamine is important for glucose metabolism; the more carbohydrate there is in the diet, the greater the need for thiamine.

One way to establish the implications of consuming a low intake of a vitamin is to feed an experimental diet that contains all other nutrients in adequate quantities but limits the provision of the vitamin in question. The first response to a thiamine-deficient diet is an inability to concentrate, confusion of thought, uncertainty of memory, anorexia, irritability and depression.[3] Following deprivation, a dose of thiamine produces dramatic changes; in particular, appetite is rapidly restored and personality changes for the better. The first signs of deficiency are likely to be psychological. A prolonged and severe deficiency can result in brain damage and even more profound cognitive changes. An interesting conclusion from one study was that it is doubtful if a minimum thiamine requirement can be meaningfully established, as there are wide individual needs.[4]

When the eating of polished rice in the Far East became widespread, it was associated with memory problems that were labelled 'beri-beri amnesia'. When the Japanese captured Singapore during the Second World War, many British soldiers became prisoners of war. As they were fed little other than polished rice, they inevitably consumed low levels of thiamine. Two doctors in the Army Medical Corps decided to carry out a scientific study.[5]

Unknown to their guards, the doctors carefully recorded changes in the prisoners; their results were hidden in a graveyard and retrieved after the war. Within six weeks the first symptoms were noticed: loss of appetite was followed by uncontrolled eye movements, sleeplessness and anxiety. Loss of memory occurred in 62 per cent of the subjects. It was the ability to store new information that was disrupted rather than the ability to recall old information. The importance of thiamine was demonstrated on the occasions when supplies of the vitamin were available. The response was dramatic and in the majority of cases the symptoms improved within two days.

In the 1940s Ruth Harrell, working at Columbia University, New York, examined 120 children who lived in the Presbyterian Orphans' Home at Lynchburg, Virginia.[6] In fact, they lived on a farm and they all ate the same diet. Following analysis at the university, it was calculated that the diet supplied 1 mg of thiamine a day. The British figures recommend a daily intake of 0.9 mg of thiamine a day for boys, and 0.7 mg for girls. So according to conventional nutritional wisdom, the diet supplied an adequate amount of thiamine. Under a double-blind procedure the children took either a placebo or 2 mg of thiamine each day for a year. There were remarkable improvements in those taking the thiamine; they were significantly taller, had better eyesight, quicker reaction times, and scored better on tests of memory and intelligence (Table 9.1). Thus we have a group of children whose intake of thiamine, as judged by traditional nutritional standards, was adequate. When they received thiamine that theoretically they did not need, they grew taller and were more intellectually able.

At the other end of the age range 48 per cent of a group of women over the age of 65 living in Cork were found to be thiamine deficient and a further 17 per cent were found to have only marginal stores. They were all apparently healthy and lived independently. When they were given daily supplements of thiamine (12.5 × RDA) for six weeks, there was a measurable improvement in their mood.[7] Other examples of poor mood being associated with low thiamine status are described in Chapter 11.

*Table 9.1* Thiamine supplementation of children

| Characteristic | Percentage of change over 1 year | |
| --- | --- | --- |
|  | *Control* | *Thiamine* |
| Height | + 1.5 | + 1.8 |
| Visual acuity | + 7.5 | + 14.0 |
| Memory of Morse Code | + 13.2 | + 30.8 |
| Memory of word/number pairs | + 20.6 | + 35.6 |
| Intelligence | + 2.8 | + 5.9 |

*Source:* Data from R. F. Harrell, *Journal of Nutrition*, 1946, 31, 283–98.

## Alcohol amnesia syndrome

Wernicke's disease is a disorder of the brain caused by thiamine deficiency; sufferers are uncoordinated, confused and have memory problems. If a person needs to be fed by an intravenous glucose drip in hospital for several days, the drip must also supply thiamine. If by mistake thiamine is missing from the drip, then memory problems will result quickly.[8] In such cases the small stores of thiamine in the body are rapidly depleted because they are needed to help the body metabolize the glucose. Treatment with thiamine will result in a complete recovery.

Korsakoff's psychosis is characterized by an inability to form new long-term memories, combined with minor intellectual impairment. If Korsakoff's patients are told a telephone number, they will be able to repeat it. As long as they are able to say it over and over again, they will be able to recall the number. If their attention is directed to something else, then they will forget the number. If they hear the number day after day, they will not learn it. They will be able to talk readily about events that occurred many years previously; their problem is in forming new memories.

In developed countries the nutritional complications associated with alcoholism are the most common cause of Korsakoff's dementia, although symptoms may result from an inability of the gut to absorb thiamine. Often the disorder is brought about by a particularly heavy drinking bout lasting two weeks or longer during which little food is eaten. Twenty-five per cent of Korsakoff's patients recover completely when treated with thiamine, and 50 per cent recover partially.[9] More recently it has become clear that Wernicke's disease and Korsakoff's syndrome represent different stages of the same disorder, the Wernicke–Korsakoff syndrome, or alcohol amnesia syndrome.

When people who have had the alcohol amnesia syndrome are examined at post-mortem, there is characteristic brain damage. It is interesting to look, at post-mortem, at the brains of individuals who were not diagnosed as having the alcohol amnesia syndrome while they were alive. The impression is gained that a deficiency of thiamine, sufficient to damage the brain, is more common in the general population than initially thought. In an Australian survey evidence of brain damage caused by a lack of thiamine was present in 2.8 per cent of the population.[10] It was concluded that only 20 per cent of those people suffering brain damage were diagnosed during life,

---

### Melanie: a girl who always felt tired

Melanie was nearly 8 when she was seen by a new paediatrician at the local hospital. She complained of feeling tired and that she readily fell asleep in class. Her sleep was restless, she snored loudly, and talked and walked in her sleep. Her heart rate was 150 beats a minute when it was taken by the paediatrician, she had a fever and sweated excessively, and her knee reflex was unpredictable. The paediatrician took a blood sample and asked for thiamine status to be established. When the test came back from the laboratory, it was clear that Melanie had a thiamine deficiency. She began taking a supplement of thiamine hydrochloride and seventeen days later she had ceased to snore, her appetite had improved and she no longer felt tired. After a month her weight had increased by 1 kg (2.2 lb) and she felt well. Her mother was advised to try to decrease the proportion of the calories consumed by Melanie that came in the form of sugar.

---

although early treatment with thiamine would have resulted in complete recovery. Such is the concern in Australia about the association between the intake of alcohol and brain damage caused by thiamine deficiency that there have been calls for action. Surprisingly, the call is not to decrease the intake of alcohol but to fortify beer with thiamine![11]

Two American researchers, Derrick Lonsdale and Raymond Shamburger, examined twenty patients who, as judged from blood samples, had low levels of thiamine. Insomnia and restless sleeping were common and the patients were aggressive and hostile. Some had physical symptoms, commonly chest pains and fever. Treatment with thiamine improved the symptoms, although the patients had previously failed to respond to psychiatric drugs or psychotherapy. The researchers described one case:

A thirteen and a half year old boy experienced violent and unpredictable mood changes for seven years. Stomach cramps, severe enough to simulate appendicitis, nervous throat clearing, intermittent diarrhea, severe episodes of depression, insomnia and frightening dreams were common symptoms. He admitted to snacking on high calorie junk foods . . . thiamin was in the deficiency range.[12]

The diet of these twenty patients was unusual in that in many, but not all, cases they ate almost exclusively large amounts of 'junk food'. Any food that contains high levels of sugar will use up the body's supply of thiamine. (It is ironic that somebody researching the impact of 'junk food' should be called Shamburger.)

If a low intake of any vitamin is going to have psychological consequences, then thiamine is the first case that should be considered. The high demand for thiamine when glucose is broken down and the relatively limited stores in the body make it reasonable to ask whether minor deficiencies may arise. A diet lacking thiamine rapidly induces a deficiency that has adverse psychological consequences. Such a diet is unusual; nobody is likely to eat anything that even approaches a deprivation diet. A low intake of thiamine over an extended period can, however, gradually deplete the body of the vitamin.

In both clinical cases and double-blind studies changes in

mood and personality have been described that were associated with a low intake of thiamine; in turn these responded to thiamine supplementation. It seems reasonable to conclude that there are some people in the population whose marginal intake of thiamine influences their psychological functioning. As always, the problem is in establishing who is and who is not marginally deficient. Table 2.4 reports that 23 per cent of a sample of young British males and 20 per cent of young British females had either marginal or deficient thiamine status. It should not, however, be assumed that such measures necessarily predict psychological functioning, as the cut-off values were created to prevent biological rather than psychological problems. Of 172 patients who were admitted to a British psychiatric hospital, 30 per cent were thiamine deficient.[13] It seems probable that in most cases there was a dietary problem because of the mental illness. There is no suggestion that solving a minor nutritional deficiency would cure mental illness, although it is likely to have helped in a small way.

## Riboflavin

Vitamin $B_2$, or riboflavin, is widely distributed in leafy vegetables, meat and fish, and the intake must be low for months before signs of deficiency appear. There is little reason to think that a deficiency of riboflavin commonly influences psychological functioning. When an extreme deficiency was created by an experimental diet almost totally lacking riboflavin, depression resulted after fifty days.[14] When the riboflavin status of those entering a British psychiatric hospital was examined, 29 per cent were found to be riboflavin deficient, particularly those suffering with depression. Although nobody suggests that vitamin deficiency is commonly the sole cause of depression, the researchers argued that it was likely that riboflavin deficiency predisposed people towards such problems. The alternative explanation is that those who become depressed stop eating a good diet.[15] Both are possible explanations of the finding.

## Niacin

Nicotinic acid and nicotinamide are the active forms of niacin, another B vitamin. An inadequate intake of niacin is associated with the deficiency disease pellagra, which is characterized by the three 'D's: dermatitis, diarrhoea and dementia. Before the physical symptoms appear there are psychological problems, including anxiety, depression and fatigue. Memory problems are a major symptom that responds to the administration of the vitamin. The possibility that minor deficiencies might occur in industrialized societies has attracted little attention. However, a niacin supplement (8 × RDA) improved the memory of healthy volunteers eating their usual diet. Thus the possibility that minor deficiencies may occur should not be discounted.[16] However, as there is no other evidence on the topic, no conclusion is warranted until more information becomes available.

The most commonly suggested benefit of niacin supplementation is that it may help schizophrenics. Schizophrenia is a label given to a group of severe forms of mental illness. The symptoms vary but include: thought disorders – sentences may be grammatical although they make little sense; delusions; hallucinations; and disturbed mood. A major theory is that the disorder results from abnormalities of the brain's chemistry.

One view is that the brain produces an abnormal chemical that is similar in structure to a hallucinogenic drug. It has been hypothesized that free methyl groups ($CH_3$) are added to naturally occurring brain chemicals, producing an abnormal chemical similar in structure to hallucinogenic drugs such as mescaline (Figure 9.1). If this were occurring, then niacin would help schizophrenics because it would mop up the methyl groups, and remove one of the building blocks from which the mescaline-like chemical was made. Today this is not the major theory of the biochemical basis of schizophrenia, but in the 1950s it attracted attention. Later, the reason for giving large doses of the vitamin was that there was said to be a niacin deficiency, at least in the brain.

Two Canadian psychologists, Abram Hoffer and Humphrey

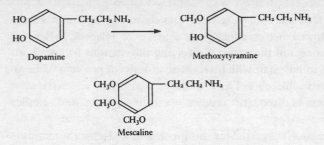

*Figure 9. 1* **Do some brains produce hallucinogenic chemicals?**
Several drugs that produce hallucinations have a structure similar to
chemicals that occur naturally in the brain. One example is dopamine,
thought to be important in the disorder schizophrenia. When dopamine is
naturally broken down in the brain, it is transformed into methoxytyramine.
Even a non-chemist can see the similarity between the structure of these
chemicals and mescaline, a drug that produces hallucinations. Is it possible
that an abnormal pathway converts dopamine into a hallucinogenic drug?
Although not now the favoured explanation of the cause of schizophrenia,
at one time the possibility was considered seriously.

Osmond, were the first to use niacin to treat schizophrenia. One
striking success was a 17-year-old girl.

Her mind was full of random thoughts which greatly troubled her. She was
diagnosed early schizophrenia and started on nicotinamide, three grams per
day. There was slight improvement . . . but on February 17, 1966, she was
worse again. She had seen a visual hallucination of a man who looked like a
Beatle (English version). For a while he was real, then vanished and she was
left confused and depressed. The medication was changed to nicotinic acid,
three grams per day, and NAD, one gram.

February 24th she was amazingly improved. She was happy, relaxed
and found it easy to talk. She reported her mind lost its fog one hour after
taking one gram of NAD . . . The NAD ran out on February 28th and she
quickly relapsed. She was started on nicotinic acid, three grams, thiamin
one hundred and fifty milligrams and riboflavin thirty milligrams per day.
On April 4th she was much better again and felt free of depression, but her
mind was still foggy. Only the NAD had cleared the fog. In September
1966, she was finally normal.[17]

The beneficial effect was confirmed when patients were followed up. Over the following two years those who had received the vitamin showed better adjustment and fewer relapses. After ten years 75 per cent of the patients receiving the vitamins had not been readmitted to hospital, which was true of only 36 per cent of those who received a placebo. These findings were taken very seriously, but a dozen subsequent studies were unable to find similar results.[18]

One reason suggested for this inconsistency is that the attempts to replicate the beneficial effect were made using long-term schizophrenics, whereas the original observations had been made on patients at an early stage of a disorder that gets progressively worse with time.

There are still some people who argue that the possibility that megadoses may be of value should not be finally discounted. It is a common idea that schizophrenia is not one disorder but several; if so, it should not be expected that all patients will respond to the same treatment. It has been proposed that niacin should be used in combination with other vitamins. Some doctors hold the view that niacin should not replace drug therapy but complement it. The American Psychiatric Association reviewed these possibilities and, in the light of a string of negative findings, opposed the therapy:

The claims of the advocates of megavitamin therapy have not been confirmed . . . It is suspected that a substantial number of patients for whom the best results are obtained may not actually have been schizophrenic and represent a group for whom spontaneous recovery is high . . . the possibility of a small subgroup that is responsive appears to be miminal.[19]

The megavitamin approach has reached an unsatisfactory position. The information from double-blind studies strongly suggests that schizophrenics in general do not respond to a high intake of vitamins, yet there are impressive claims that particular individuals respond. People taking the orthomolecular approach will claim that the vitamin supplements need to be tailored to the needs of the individual. Thus the double-blind approach of giving everybody the same doses of the same vitamins is inappropriate. Individuals using the orthomolecular approach refuse to use a rigorous scientific method of evaluation, and traditional scientists simply refuse to consider the idea further. A possibility that is worthy of consideration is that there is a subgroup of people who are amenable to dietary treatment. Without hard evidence this possibility will never be taken seriously.

## Vitamin B₆

A gross deficiency of vitamin $B_6$ may cause weakness, difficulty in walking, loss of a sense of responsibility, insomnia and depression.[20] The impact of vitamin $B_6$ supplements on psychological functioning has been little studied and the few attempts that have been made have resulted in negative findings.[21] Elderly people are at a particularly high risk of vitamin deficiency, as their physiology is increasingly inefficient and they are more likely to consume inadequate meals. For these reasons a group of Dutch researchers gave vitamin $B_6$ (14 × RDA) to men who were over 70 years of age and found that their long-term memory improved.[22]

### Autism

Autism is one of the most severe psychiatric disorders of children. A child with autism will often appear normal until language begins to develop. Parents begin to become concerned when they notice that their child is acting as if they do not exist. Such children use words, but not as a means of communication; people are treated in a similar manner to other objects. Eye contact is not made and there is an aversion to being touched. The disorder clearly reflects significant brain damage. Although autistic children have intellectual problems, these may not be uniform; in fact, they may have some unusual gift. Some combine a supra-normal ability with a lack of abilities in other areas. The term 'idiot savant' is used, although with the rise of political correctness this sounds dated. One individual may be able to draw from memory a Gothic cathedral that has been viewed only once. Others may be able to perform amazing feats of memory or calculation, although they are unable to spell or read. For example, in one case there was an ability to calculate the day of the week on which a particular date fell. You try to work out in a few minutes on which day of the week 19 August 1876 fell.

Autistic children are in many cases unable to metabolize the amino acid tryptophan in a normal manner. In the 1960s two English doctors examined nineteen autistic children and found that eleven displayed this problem.[23] When these eleven were given 30 mg of vitamin B$_6$ their bodies began to deal with tryptophan in a normal manner. The vitamin B$_6$ was administered on only one occasion as part of this biochemical experiment. No attempt was made by the researchers to take this observation further. One parent, Professor Jeremy Noakes, did, however, follow up the finding and later wrote to the *Observer* newspaper, describing the result.

Our child was diagnosed as autistic by two different specialists at the age of two-and-a-half and went into hospital for a year, though he came home at weekends. A biochemical test showed that he lacked Pyridoxine (Vitamin B$_6$). A number of other autistic children were tested at the same time and the same was found to be true of some of them, though not of all. Since then we have been giving him the vitamin daily in pill-form. About three months after we started, he said his first word (Bus!). Since then his improvement had been rapid and steady. He now has a vocabulary of approximately 400 words, he can use short sentences to express his wants and observations, understands the use of letters and numbers, and above all is beginning to appreciate other people. He will be five in December. His behaviour is still autistic in many ways, but his progress, judged by any standards, seems remarkable.[24]

The findings of such case studies need to be followed up, but offer little more than an interesting idea requiring more systematic study. It is unclear whether the improvement, which was not complete, would have occurred without the vitamin simply because the boy was growing older. More systematic evidence was, however, being collected.

Bernard Rimland is Director of the Institute for Child Behavior Research in San Diego. For many years he has been a powerful advocate the orthomolecular approach to childhood disorders. In the 1960s there was a climate that encouraged the taking of large doses of vitamins for a range of disorders. In the absence of knowledge or theory parents tried many combinations of vitamins, in a range of doses, with little more than hope to guide them. Bernard Rimland systematically obtained reports from parents who did, or did not, find that their child's autistic symptoms improved. When all these data were placed in a computer, it was found that when an improvement was reported, the giving of vitamin $B_6$ seemed to be the common factor. As the giving of other vitamins was not associated with a similar improvement, it was argued that the effect was more than a placebo response. The observation was confirmed using a double-blind procedure.[25] The conclusion that some autistic children respond to vitamin $B_6$ has been supported in a series of small-scale studies by teams in Tours, France, and the Langley Porter Institute in San Francisco using up to 1 g of vitamin $B_6$ (1,000 × RDA).[26] Usually magnesium is also administered to decrease side effects such as irritability, sound sensitivity and enuresis. It appears that not all autistic children benefit; usually only about one-third to one-half respond.

Bernard Rimland describes how on one occasion he was introduced by the chair of a scientific conference in Venezuela.

In introducing me, Dr Negron explained that some time earlier she had been approached by a weeping mother of an 18-year-old autistic man. The patient was extremely aggressive and had been forced to leave two psychiatric hospitals because the staff could not manage him. Various drugs had been tried, at high dosage levels, but to no avail. He was now residing in a third psychiatric institution and was considered so dangerous and difficult to manage that he was about to be evicted from this third, and last, facility.

The mother was at her wits' end and came to Dr Negron in despair. Since a variety of drugs had been tried and proven ineffective, Dr Negron had little to offer until she remembered about the work with vitamin $B_6$. She tried vitamin $B_6$ on the young man, with quite remarkable results.

The autistic young man improved so much that it was soon possible for him to leave the institution and live at home. Dr Negron had visited the town where her patient and his family lived. She had a most enjoyable visit, and was especially pleased to tell the audience that the autistic patient had been discovered to have musical talent. He played the guitar and sang for Dr Negron.[27]

The benefits most frequently observed are an increased use of sounds, better sleep, better attention and decreased hyperactivity. High doses of vitamin $B_6$ should be administered with care, as there are reports that 0.5 g of vitamin $B_6$ a day can cause nerve damage, resulting in numbness in the fingers and an unsteady walk.[28] Photosensitive blisters have also been reported in children. However, in many trials no side effects have been reported or they were minor enough to be discounted. Parents typically report that the benefits outweigh the costs.

The use of megavitamins is controversial and the possibility of alternative approaches should be fully considered. Medicine is a conservative profession and the use of vitamin $B_6$ for the treatment of autistic children is not widely accepted. Yet the evidence suggests that we should consider seriously the possibility of a beneficial response to vitamin $B_6$. Positive findings from a large-scale trial would increase the confidence that could be placed in the finding. Although there are an increasing number of positive reports from the researchers in Tours, France, it is unclear how many children have been studied. The use of vitamin $B_6$ to treat autism raises many as yet unanswered questions.

Parents who have autistic children and are interested in the vitamin $B_6$ approach should discuss it with their doctor, rather than introducing the treatment themselves. Their doctor might consider it and possibly integrate it with other approaches. Any adverse reactions that occur should be monitored.

## Vitamin C

Many vegetables and fruits contain vitamin C, or ascorbic acid. The clinical description of the deficiency disorder scurvy includes behavioural symptoms such as fatigue, apathy and weakness. Similarly, experimentally induced scurvy increases reaction times, fatigue,[29] anxiety and depression.[30] It should be remembered that these symptoms appear only after several months of an extremely low intake of vitamin C. There is little evidence that levels associated with typical diets in industrialized societies are likely to be so low that they would have psychological consequences. An exception is the observation that the intelligence scores of those with low blood levels of vitamin C increased when given orange juice, something that did not occur in those with adequate bodily supplies.[31] The possibility that low vitamin C status is associated with poorer intellectual ability was supported by the finding that they were correlated: children with higher levels of vitamin C tended to have higher intelligence scores.[32] Given the little information available, it is unreasonable to definitely conclude that minor deficiencies of vitamin C disrupt us psychologically but the possibility should not be discarded.

There is more reason to suggest that high doses of vitamin C may have some pharmacological action; in particular, that they influence the functioning of dopamine, a chemical in the brain that plays an important role in controlling mood.[33] In normal subjects large doses of vitamin C (50 × RDA) depressed reaction times and coordination:[34] there is no rule that says that vitamin supplements can have only positive consequences. Psychiatric patients given vitamin C (25 or 75 × RDA) for three weeks were less depressed.[35] There is, however, no suggestion that vitamin C offers an alternative to traditional antidepressant drugs. Rather than there being any nutritional explanation for the findings, it is likely that large doses of vitamin C have a weak drug-like action.

## Multivitamin supplements and learning disabilities

Learning disabilities can exist for a range of reasons, but, unlike autism, the intellectual deficits are more uniform and the peculiar emotional disturbance of autism is lacking.

There are several clinical reports that the administration of vitamin and mineral supplements benefits children with learning disabilities. For example, an American paediatrician reported that he had successfully treated 500 children, with varying degrees of learning disabilities, with high doses of vitamins C (33 × RDA), B$_6$ (200–400 × RDA) and niacin (85–170 × RDA).[36] Although sometimes dramatic improvements in learning ability were claimed, as these were case reports rather than experimental observations, we should look for more reliable data.

In 1981 Ruth Harrell attracted the attention of both the scientific community and the parents of children with learning disabilities. She described a 7-year-old boy who, when initially seen, was in nappies, could not speak, and whose estimated intelligence was under 30. When a nutritional supplement was given, there was no noticeable result for several weeks, but when the levels of some of the constituents were increased (eleven vitamins 4–700 × RDA plus eight minerals) there was a sudden and dramatic improvement.

In a few days he was talking a little; in a few weeks he was learning to read and write, and began to act like a normal child. When he was nine years old he read and wrote on the elementary school level, was moderately advanced in arithmetic, and, according to his teacher, was mischievous and active. He rode a bicycle and a skate board, played ball, played a flute and had an IQ of about 90.[37]

This remarkable case stimulated a double-blind trial using children with learning disabilities (IQ 17–70). The intelligence scores of the five receiving the supplement increased significantly more than the scores of those who received the placebo. When those who had initially received the placebo were subsequently given the vitamin–mineral tablet, their intelligence scores increased by at least 10.2 points, although this second stage was not double-blind.[38] After eight months of supplementation one 5-year-old, who previously could say only single words such as 'Mama' or 'bye-bye', could recite, without prompting, the American Pledge of Allegiance and could read a book designed for 6-year-old pupils.

Unfortunately, the same pattern as with niacin and schizophrenia unfolded. About ten studies further examined the influence of supplements but could find no significant improvement.[39] Those people who take the 'genetotrophic' approach are not impressed by such studies and argue that the sweeping generalization that megavitamins are ineffective is not warranted. The 'genetotrophic' approach implies that, for genetic reasons, an afflicted person requires a high intake of a specific nutrient. What that specific nutrient is differs from person to person. It follows that supplements have to be tailored to individual needs: it is inappropriate to give the same supplement to everybody. Supporters of this approach would say that learning disabilities can reflect a range of aberrant mechanisms, and that there is a need to establish the efficacy, or otherwise, of giving a variety of supplements to particular subgroups. Children need to be carefully described in terms of both behavioural and biochemical parameters; nobody believes that all will respond in a similar manner.

A more specific suggestion is that Down's syndrome is associated with a deficiency of vitamin $B_6$. In Ruth Harrell's study she noted that children with Down's syndrome were the only ones whose physical appearance changed notably; they tended to lose the fluid that had accumulated in their faces and extremities. The largest gain in IQ, 25 points, was found in a Down's syndrome patient. These findings led to the impact of megavitamins on patients with Down's syndrome being examined specifically, and a series of double-blind studies followed.[40] Unfortunately, the conclusion that a broad range of megavitamins does not improve the functioning of children with Down's syndrome now seems inevitable. Yet very substantial changes were initially reported and there remains the hope that a particular factor may be found that distinguishes a subgroup that responds to supplementation. Such a hope is, however, perhaps optimistic.

### Hyperactivity

The megavitamin approach has also been taken with hyperactive children. An early attempt was made to achieve the orthomolecular psychiatry goal of matching the provision of micronutrients to the needs of the child. Children were exposed to various substances on different days (143 × RDA thiamine, 300 × RDA vitamin $B_6$, 32 × RDA calcium); only if there was a response was a placebo trial instituted. Of 100 hyperactive children, 11 dramatically responded to thiamine and got worse when the placebo was administered, 4 similarly responded to calcium and 9 to vitamin $B_6$ There was no suggestion that all children responded to supplementation, although 24 per cent did respond.[41] As the trial was not double-blind, a large placebo response could be expected, and the data should be treated with caution.

## The safety of supplementation

Some people seem to believe that because vitamins are 'natural chemicals' they can be taken safely in large doses. As some of the most poisonous substances known are 'natural', this does not follow logically.

Low doses of vitamins – that is, food supplements – are so safe that they are freely available in supermarkets, and are classified in Britain not as drugs but as foods. Clearly, this would not occur unless they were very safe to take at the doses recommended (about 1 × RDA). In contrast, some of the doses that have been used to manipulate behaviour are vastly in excess of the RDA (up to 1,000 × RDA). Even if essential for life in low doses, it does not necessarily follow that high doses are safe. In fact, there is little doubt that taking high doses of some, but not all, vitamins can cause problems.

John Marks, the Director of Medical Studies at Girton College, Cambridge, suggested that vitamins can be split into two groups:[42] those, including most but not all the water-soluble vitamins, that can safely be taken in doses at least 50 to 100 times the RDA; and those with a safety ratio of about ten times the RDA that should be administered at higher doses only under medical supervision. The toxicity of the fat-soluble vitamins A and D is well documented.

For a long time water-soluble vitamins were considered to be nontoxic; it was assumed that any excess was simply excreted in the urine. The report that vitamin $B_6$ (30 × RDA) can produce nerve damage has been the cause of concern,[43] although a comprehensive review of the safety of this vitamin concluded that lesser doses appear to be safe.[44]

The side-effects of niacin (3 × RDA) include flushing and headaches, although nicotinamide is free of these effects. A number of disorders, such as asthma, diabetes mellitus and peptic ulcers, may be aggravated by a large dose of niacin. In the late 1980s the use of high doses of niacin became a fashionable way to reduce cholesterol levels. In 1990 the *Journal of the American Medical Association* reported how a 20-year-old man developed hepatitis a week after starting to take 6 g of niacin a day. Immediately he stopped taking the vitamin he recovered. There have been reports of death due to liver damage following the taking of niacin (175–350 × RDA).

Although there has also been concern about kidney problems following the taking of gram quantities of vitamin C (40 × RDA), a reviewer concluded that 'the consensus . . . is that these adverse effects are not induced in healthy persons'.[45]

In the light of the known adverse reactions to large doses of a few vitamins, and the cautious position that as yet unsuspected side-effects may become apparent, it seems sensible to suggest that megavitamin therapy should be implemented only under medical supervision. In most cases a decision to take the megavitamin approach reflects hope rather than reasonable expectation. The possibility should always be considered that there are other treatments available with a greater likelihood of success.

Perhaps part of the heat of the debate generated by megavitamins reflects the way that the desperate parents of hyperactive, autistic or schizophrenic children turn to practitioners of fringe medicine. To attract patients, it may be tempting for such practitioners to overstate their case, either knowingly or perhaps more frequently because of a deep belief that the approach has much to offer. A vicious circle is created whereby unconventional ideas are given an even worse name by unscrupulous practitioners. The history of the area is of megadoses of vitamins initially offering great hope that turns out to be only false promise. As this sequence has been repeated on several occasions, it is inevitable that any new claim is greeted with scepticism.

# CHAPTER 10

# Can Diet Slow Ageing?

In the West death is increasingly viewed as defeat: if you do not live to be 100, then it must reflect some self-inflicted injury. Clearly, lifestyle has much to do with life expectancy. Whether you smoke, whether you exercise and the nature of your diet are ways in which you can influence how long you live.

In considering sections of industrialized societies that have a poor diet, the elderly are a high-risk group. There are a number of potential problems that arise with increasing age. Physical problems such as the loss of teeth may make the eating of some foods difficult. Arthritis may make walking around shops difficult, and the preparation of food may be similarly affected. Elderly people may be short of money, limiting the range of foods bought. Illness may prevent shopping and limit the ability to cook. When a partner dies, the survivor may lose the motivation to cook only for him- or herself. If the partner who had traditionally done the cooking dies, the survivor may lack the basic knowledge and experience to provide an adequate diet. With age, the body absorbs nutrients from food less efficiently.

The major diet-related problem of old age is obesity. As people become less active, they consume too many calories. However, surveys of the micronutrient intake of elderly people regularly provide evidence of deficiencies of ascorbic acid, folic acid and iron. In a survey of elderly people in Britain 3.2 per cent were described as malnourished.[1] Out of 879, 2 had scurvy and 8 were excessively thin. If the diet of some was so bad that it caused clinical problems, then many can be expected to have more minor deficiencies. Intakes of vitamins and minerals that are below the recommended levels are common, although as we learnt in Chapter 2 this is not evidence that there is necessarily a problem. A review of studies of the nutritional status of elderly people in the United States commented that unmistakable vitamin deficiencies are seen rarely, although it is common to find dietary intakes of the water-soluble B vitamins below the recommended levels.[2]

A group of American geriatricians related vitamin status and cognitive functioning in elderly people.[3] They found that those with higher levels of folic acid, riboflavin, and vitamins C and $B_{12}$ had a better memory. Higher levels of riboflavin and folic acid were also positively related to the ability to think abstractly. An interesting aspect of this finding is that the subjects were healthy, affluent, middle-class Americans living in their own homes. They were not individuals who were obviously at high risk of dietary problems. Although such a finding alerts us to a potential problem, all we have is a correlation. It may be that those subjects with better vitamin status were generally more health orientated. Did they eat better, take more exercise and were they less likely to smoke and drink alcohol? If so, a better vitamin status would simply be indicative of a more healthy lifestyle; we would be unable to say which parts of that lifestyle resulted in better memory. Was it the diet that was important or something else? As is often the case, the crucial evidence we look for comes from studies that have administered vitamin supplements under double-blind conditions. Such studies are few and far between, although there are suggestions that poor vitamin status may, on occasions, be the cause of problems. In Bristol 90 per cent of an elderly population had low levels of thiamine and vitamin C. The giving of a complex of B vitamins and vitamin C improved both their physical and mental abilities, although in some cases the changes took a year to develop.[4] Thiamine supplementation improved the mood of elderly women in Cork, Ireland.[5]

## Vitamin $B_{12}$

Vitamin $B_{12}$ is necessary for the formation of the oxygen-carrying red blood cells. It is required by the body in very small amounts and body stores will last several years. When it is absent from the diet or poorly absorbed by the gut, pernicious anaemia results. Clinically, a lack of vitamin $B_{12}$ is characterized by pallor, a prolonged bleeding time, loss of weight, abdominal discomfort and loss of appetite. There are also profound effects on the nervous system. Initially, there may be numbness and tingling of the hands and feet. Later, there are problems associated with the brain, including confusion, problems of memory, moodiness, delusions and hallucinations, all of which respond rapidly to treatment with vitamin $B_{12}$. As vitamin $B_{12}$ is found almost exclusively in food from animal sources, vegans, who consume no dairy products, eggs or meat, are likely to be deficient unless they take supplements. Generally, however, a vitamin $B_{12}$ deficiency due to inadequate intake is very rare; problems with its absorption are more likely.

It is standard medical practice, when faced with an elderly person displaying psychological problems, to take a blood sample and measure vitamin $B_{12}$ and folic acid levels. Numerous investigators have reported associations between deficiencies of vitamins $B_{12}$ and folic acid and psychiatric symptoms including depression and dementia.[6] Some think that cognitive impairment, hallucinations and delusions are particularly associated with $B_{12}$ deficiency.[7]

## Folic acid

Folic acid was discovered in the 1930s when scientists were looking for the factor in the liver that cured pernicious anaemia. Although folic acid stimulated the regeneration of red blood cells, it did not solve the neurological problems associated with pernicious anaemia. Subsequently, it was found that vitamin $B_{12}$ was the true anti-pernicious-anaemia factor and that folic acid was necessary for normal cell division.

Folic acid deficiency is common in people with diseases of the digestive tract, in alcoholics and in elderly people with a limited intake of fruit and vegetables. There is increasing evidence that folic acid deficiency may influence behaviour, in particular psychiatric symptoms, including irritability, hostility and paranoia. In elderly psychiatric patients a low folic acid level is associated with more severe symptoms[8] than in younger individuals; these may even occur when the levels of folic acid are acceptable according to traditional definitions. It is thought that in elderly people depression is particularly associated with folic acid deficiency.[9]

There is little doubt that on occasion a low vitamin level can be the cause of psychological problems in elderly people. It should not, however, be assumed that vitamin deficiencies occur frequently or that they are the only cause of any particular problem.

## Alzheimer's disease

Every year apparently healthy individuals in their 40s and 50s begin to lose the ability to name familiar people and objects or to find the correct word. They look well and there is no obvious physical problem, such as a brain tumour or stroke. Within three to ten years they will be severely demented, unable to speak or take care of themselves. They are not displaying the normal characteristics of ageing, but have a disorder first described by Alois Alzheimer, a German neurologist, in 1860. Table 10.1 summarizes the changes observed in this very unpleasant disorder, which is known as Alzheimer's disease.

The disorder starts with difficulties in concentrating, absent-mindedness and irritability. The individual tends to blame other people for the consequences of these problems and may have delusions of being persecuted. As memory continues to deteriorate, the individual becomes increasingly agitated and disorientated. The disorder is disturbing for the family, as, to a large extent, we are our memories; our personality reflects a lifetime of experiences. As the memory fails, the personality inevitably changes. Judged by their personality, people with Alzheimer's are not the individuals their family and friends have known and loved, although physically they appear to be the same. It is inevitably upsetting if, for example, individuals are unable to recognize their spouse or children. The ability to write, read and even speak in an intelligent manner may be forgotten. If the disorder appears prior to 60 years of age, it is described as Alzheimer's disease. If it occurs after this age, it is

*Table 10.1* **Progression of Alzheimer's disease**

|  | *Stage one:* 1–3 years | *Stage two:* 2–10 years | *Stage three:* 8–12 years |
|---|---|---|---|
| Memory | Remote memory impaired | Recent and remote memory impaired | Severely deteriorated |
| Language | Difficulty finding words | Incomprehensible speech | Severely deteriorated |
| Personality | Apathy, irritability | Indifference | Severely deteriorated |
| Visuo–spatial | Inability to reproduce simple pattern | Well-executed but incorrect movements | Severely deteriorated |

known as Senile Dementia of Alzheimer's Type. About one in ten people over 65, and one in five over 80 years, have a dementia, of which about three-quarters are Alzheimer's. About 2 million Americans are estimated to have this complaint.

When the brains of Alzheimer's patients are examined after death, the presence of so-called senile plaques throughout the cerebral cortex is noticeable. The cerebral cortex is the area of the brain most developed in humans; it is thought to play a major role in allowing humans to perform the intellectual tasks that distinguish them from other animals. Senile plaques are small round areas in which the tissue has degenerated. Tangled threadlike structures (neurofibrillary tangles) replace normal nerve cells. As a high concentration of aluminium is found in the senile plaques, the possibility that alumunium in the diet influences the development of the disorder has been considered.

## Aluminium

In an ageing population the suggestion that aluminium may cause Alzheimer's disease has received a great deal of attention. It has led to suggestions that aluminium cooking utensils and cooking foil should be thrown away. It is inevitable that small amounts of aluminium from a pan will be deposited in food while cooking. To what extent is this concern well founded?

There are four lines of evidence that have caused aluminium to be viewed with suspicion. Firstly, the post-mortem brains of Alzheimer's patients have high levels of aluminium concentrated in those areas of the brain that have degenerated. However, in itself this does not prove that aluminium caused the brain damage. Possibly the disease occurs and at a later stage aluminium is concentrated in the brain. By whatever means it enters the brain, there is widespread agreement that aluminium is present in toxic concentration in the brains of Alzheimer's patients.

Secondly, aluminium injected into the brains of animals produces changes that are similar to those found in the brains of people suffering with Alzheimer's disease. The ability of these animals in learning tasks is poorer after an aluminium injection. However, although aluminium damages the animals' brains, the changes are not identical to those seen in the brains of Alzheimer's patients. These differences are important and suggest that aluminium is not the simple cause of the disorder. At the very least, some other mechanism is also involved.

There is an irreversible dementia that develops in some people who have repeatedly undergone kidney dialysis using dialysis solutions that contain aluminium. The dementia associated with kidney dialysis is not, however, identical in all respects to Alzheimer's disease.

A third approach is to examine the incidence of Alzheimer's disease in different parts of the country to see if those areas where the incidence is highest also have the highest levels of aluminium in the drinking water. There have been several reports that higher levels of aluminium in the water supply are associated with a greater risk of Alzheimer's disease, although the relationship has not been found in other studies. The increased risk of Alzheimer's disease in people drinking water with high concentrations of aluminium is similar to the increased risk of lung cancer in people who work in a smoky atmosphere but are not smokers themselves. At the worst, the additional risk is small. Drinking water accounts for only a small amount of the aluminium that is consumed. Most people living in areas with high concentrations of aluminium in the water do not get Alzheimer's disease.

There is no evidence that an increase in aluminium in the brain is associated with age as such (in people without Alzheimer's disease) or that it pre-dates symptoms in people with Alzheimer's disease. One possibility is that early in Alzheimer's disease the brain starts to be permeable to aluminium. If this explanation proves to be true, then aluminium does not cause the disorder, although it may play a role in the speed of its development. Consistent with this explanation is the final line of evidence that comes from studies that have found that the use of drugs, such as desferrioxamine, that remove aluminium from the body slow the progress of the disease. Such drugs do not, however, prevent the development of the disorder, only slow it down. These drugs are at present largely experimental tools and we await a large-scale evaluation of their effectiveness.

Disorders such as Alzheimer's disease are not caused by a single factor, so it is not sensible to ask if aluminium is the single cause of the disorder. At the worst, it will prove to be one of several risk factors. As the evaluation of data such as those outlined in the preceding paragraphs is a highly technical exercise, it is not appropriate at present to examine the strengths and weaknesses of studies on which the conclusions depend. At the forefront of science, where truth has not yet been conclusively demonstrated, there is considerable room for personal opinion. The aluminium and Alzheimer's topic falls into this category.

Sir Richard Doll is the most eminent British epidemiologist, famous for the work that first associated smoking with lung cancer. After reviewing the relationship between aluminium and Alzheimer's disease, he concluded 'that aluminium is neurotoxic in humans, but not that it is a cause of Alzheimer's disease. The possibility that it is must, however, be kept open . . .'[10] For Richard Doll the evidence was not strong enough to implicate aluminium in this degenerative disorder, neither was it strong enough to totally discount the possibility. Other scientists put the stress on the other side of the equation. The leading Canadian researchers on the topic concluded: 'Taking all the evidence into account from several independent lines of investigation, it is highly probable that the toxic consequences of aluminium accumulation are involved in the Alzheimer's disease degenerative process.'[11] Again, they were not prepared to come to a definite conclusion but felt that the balance of probability was that the ingestion of aluminium should be limited, particularly in elderly people. The role of aluminium in Alzheimer's disease remains controversial.

In the advanced stages of Alzheimer's disease the provision of adequate nutrition can become a major problem. It is not uncommon to find patients who have difficulty in keeping food in the mouth. They have forgotten how to eat, and play with and refuse their food. They do not reliably communicate hunger and thirst. The problems of the disorder can be made worse by malnutrition and dehydration. For these reasons many patients benefit from dietary supplements to ensure an adequate intake of calories, vitamins and minerals.

## Should you avoid aluminium?

If you have a friend or relative with the early signs of Alzheimer's disease, what should you do? The answer that a role for aluminium in the causation of the disorder has not been definitively demonstrated is the usual 'sitting on the fence' scientific conclusion. When faced with a progressive disorder for which there is no effective treatment, you have not got time for yet more research to be painstakingly carried out. You must act immediately.

Fortunately, there is little if any evidence in the young, or in the elderly not suffering with Alzheimer's disease, that aluminium is a problem. For most of us any aluminium in our diet is very poorly absorbed. However, people with Alzheimer's disease or, more accurately, those caring for them may wish to consider decreasing contact with aluminium. In the absence of the prospect of an anti-dementia drug, a decreased exposure to aluminium offers a possible, although limited, means of helping. Some of the steps are easily taken: avoid aluminium cooking utensils, cans and foils. Do not use aluminium-based anti-perspirants, toothpastes, cosmetics, soaps and drugs, such as antacids, that contain the element. Avoid food items with high aluminium levels, such as tea. Find out if the water in your area is high in aluminium and if it is, find another source. Accept that at the most you are going to decrease the contact with aluminium and not completely avoid it. Above all, keep the role of aluminium in

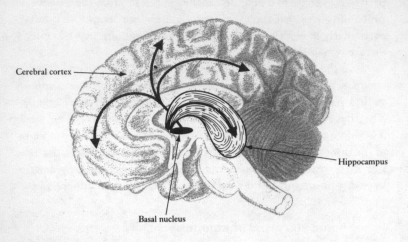

Cerebral cortex

Hippocampus

Basal nucleus

*Figure 10.1* **Alzheimer's disease and acetylcholine**
The marked pathways, which contain acetylcholine, degenerate in people
with Alzheimer's disease.

perspective. Alzheimer's disease is characterized by a progressive
decline; you will not achieve a cure. Decreasing aluminium may or
may not help, but at least it is not going to do any harm. The
thought that you may in a small way be helping will offer some
comfort, although at the most you will help only to a small
extent.

## Diet, acetylcholine and Alzheimer's disease

One hypothesis concerning the problems that cause Alzheimer's
disease is based on the observation, first made in the 1970s, that
nerve cells containing the chemical acetylcholine were particularly
likely to degenerate. Acetylcholine is a neurotransmitter, one of the
chemicals that send messages between nerve cells. Figure 10.1 illustrates the major areas of the brain that have pathways that contain
acetylcholine. It is such pathways that particularly, although not
exclusively, degenerate in Alzheimer's patients. A large loss of cells

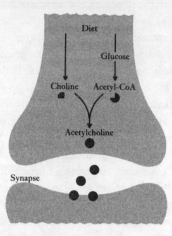

*Figure 10.2* **Formation of acetylcholine**
Acetylcholine is formed in nerve cells and released into the synapse as a
messenger that stimulates the next nerve cell. It is formed from two
chemicals, the levels of which can be increased by changing the diet.

containing acetylcholine occurs in an area deep in the brain (basal
nucleus). This area sends messages to the cortex, the area so important for thought, and to the hippocampus, which is important for
memory.

Figure 10.2 illustrates the way that acetylcholine is formed in
the brain. Two chemicals, acetyl-CoA and choline, are combined.
The supply of choline comes mainly from the diet and the acetyl-
CoA results from the breakdown of glucose, which, in part, reflects
recent food consumption. As the death of nerve cells containing
acetylcholine is a major characteristic of Alzheimer's disease, there
have been many attempts to increase the level of acetylcholine in the
brain by altering the provision of nutrients.

Attempts to help Alzheimer's patients have concentrated on
increasing the level of either acetyl-CoA or choline. It has been
suggested that an increased provision of the brain's glucose will
provide an enhanced source of acetyl-CoA. The theory behind giving
either glucose or large amounts of choline or lecithin, a complex of

choline and fatty acids, is that if the level of the raw materials is increased, the production of acetylcholine will increase.

Lecithin is found in liver, meats, fish, eggs and butter, and is used as an emulsifying agent in the manufacture of margarine and chocolate. In the human body it is part of the sheath that insulates nerve cells, and is broken down to provide choline.

Choline is the active constituent of lecithin and in this form is more easily absorbed by the body. It is a water-soluble member of the vitamin B complex. However, it is not a true vitamin in that it can be synthesized by the liver in limited quantities. Although the evidence is lacking that it is an essential part of the human diet, it seems likely that most choline in the human body is derived from diet. Foods with high concentrations of choline include liver, egg yolk, beef steak, wheat-germ and cereals. Two functions it fulfils are as part of the structure of cell membranes (as part of lecithin) and as part of the structure of acetylcholine. A problem with choline administration is that it results in foul, fishy-smelling sweat. For this and other reasons lecithin has usually been the substance of choice.

As often is the case, the initial reports suggested that Alzheimer's patients benefited from taking lecithin supplements for a short period.[12] These findings encouraged more systematic examinations of the topic, which in many cases failed to confirm the initial promise. Whether the long-term use of such dietary changes may slow the decline that inevitably occurs in this disorder awaits to be examined.

It has been suggested that there is more than one type of Alzheimer's disease; that those people who develop the disorder later in life tend to have a milder form that largely reflects a lack of acetylcholine. There are several reports that although not all Alzheimer's patients respond to either choline or lecithin, some do. It may be that those with mild cognitive impairment are more likely to respond.[13] A summary of more recent studies concluded that the results 'offer no compelling reason for the clinician to believe that Alzheimer's patients will improve significantly with choline or lecithin treatment'.[14]

## Blood glucose and acetylcholine

Glucose is the main source of the acetyl groups that are needed to create acetylcholine. In rats, if the levels of glucose in the blood are increased, the amount of glucose entering the brain increases and the rate at which acetylcholine is formed rises.[15] Therefore, if the memory problems of elderly people reflect a lack of acetylcholine in the brain, it would seem reasonable to predict that a glucose drink would improve memory. In fact, there are many reports that a glucose drink improves the memory of Alzheimer's patients.[16]

After we eat, the levels of glucose in the blood increase rapidly. The way in which the body of an elderly person deals with these rises in blood glucose predicts the individual's ability to remember.[17] If after a person eats, the blood glucose levels rise to high levels and fall only slowly, he or she is said to tolerate blood glucose poorly. Elderly people who tolerate glucose poorly have more problems of memory and attention. If when people are trying to remember something, their blood glucose falls rapidly, they tend to have a better memory. It is tempting to suggest that falling blood glucose levels in part reflect glucose being taken up by the brain. If the glucose is entering the brain, then an increased ability to synthesize acetylcholine would be expected.

Although consuming a glucose drink has been found to benefit the elderly, it does not offer an obvious means of dealing with memory problems. After a glucose drink, the levels in the blood rise rapidly but also fall rapidly. Any benefit is short lived. A diet that to a large extent contains glucose drinks is likely to produce problems. Micronutrient shortages, obesity and lack of appetite at mealtimes could all result. A logical approach would be to try to raise blood glucose levels by eating several small snacks at regular intervals rather than larger meals. Such an approach has not been examined, but it may prove to have some small benefit.

## Carnitine

Carnitine has a critical role in several aspects of energy production.[18] Animal products, particularly red meat and the whey of dairy products, are the best dietary sources of carnitine. Carnitine can, however, also be synthesized in the liver and kidney. No recommended daily amount of carnitine has been established for adults; the official line is that most well-nourished adults can probably synthesize adequate amounts.

Acetyl-carnitine is a derivative of carnitine. The treatment of ageing rats with acetyl-carnitine for six to eight months has been found to improve their ability to remember.[19] The brains of rats who have received acetyl-carnitine have fewer signs of ageing;[20] in fact, acetyl-carnitine decreases the mortality of rats.[21] Carnitine and acetylcholine have similar chemical structures.

There is a consistent finding that acetyl-carnitine improves the symptoms of people with dementia. As one example, when mildly demented elderly patients received acetyl-carnitine for three months, both their behaviour and memory improved.[22] There are a number of similar findings from small-scale double-blind studies. There is an urgent need for a large-scale study of this food derivative. Until then its value as an anti-ageing compound is uncertain; it is only an experimental drug.

## Starve yourself to a long life

It may seem obvious that a good diet will be associated with good health and a long life. Yet there is strong evidence that restricting the amount that you eat may increase your life span! Figure 10.3 illustrates data from two such experiments. Mice allowed free access to food throughout life lived for an average of twenty-seven months; those eating 25 per cent fewer calories lived for thirty-three months; and those eating 65 per cent less had an average life of forty-five months.[23] There is no reason to believe that these changes reflect an increased maximum age; rather, more animals survived to an older

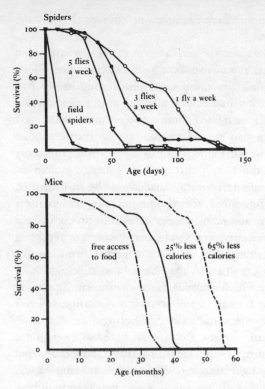

*Figure 10.3* **Food deprivation and life expectancy**
In both mice and doily spiders the restriction of food intake markedly
increased life span.
*Source:* Weindruch *et al., Journal of Nutrition,* 116, 1989, 641; Austrad,
*Experimental Gerontology,* 24, 1989, 83–92.

age within the normal life expectancy. The figure also shows that the
average life expectancy of doily spiders is about ninety days when
given one fly a week to eat, but less than sixty days when five flies
were consumed every week.[24] These findings are robust, similar
results having been observed in a wide range of species.

That the restriction of calories increases the life span of insects,
fish, worms and all mammalian species examined strongly suggests
that humans would respond similarly. In fact, it would be very

surprising if they did not. There has been one attempt to study the phenomenon in humans.[25]

Healthy subjects 72 years of age, living in a religious institution for the elderly, received one of two diets for up to three years. One group received 2,300 calories every day. The second group had 2,300 calories on one day but only 1 litre ($1\frac{3}{4}$ pints) of milk and 500 g (1lb) of fresh fruit, providing about 1,000 calories, on the next day. During the three-year period people on the restricted diet spent 123 days in the infirmary, compared with a significantly greater 219 days for those in the control group. Six people on restricted diets died, compared with thirteen on the control diet. Although apparently consistent with the proposition that eating a little less is good for you, a single report is unlikely to convince a sceptical scientist. Obviously, everybody knew who was receiving particular diets, and, inevitably, whether a person went to the infirmary involved judgement that may have been subconsciously influenced by knowing which diet was being consumed. The more objective measure, death, was in the predicted direction, but not quite different enough to be statistically significant.

At first glance it may appear that actuarial tables may produce evidence against the proposition. Life-insurance tables show that underweight people have the highest level of mortality; being slightly overweight is associated with the greatest life expectancy. These problems may be more apparent than real. There is, for example, a much higher incidence of smoking in underweight people; it may be that they are underweight because they smoke. More importantly, the weights collected by life insurance companies do not reflect attempts to restrict calorie intake. These individuals are not underweight because they are restricting their calorie input; the largest single factor determining weight is likely to be genetic.

There have been systematic attempts to establish the means by which the restriction of diet increases life expectancy. The procedure has been summarized as 'undernutrition without malnutrition'. It is important to distinguish malnutrition in non-industrialized countries, where a lack of calories is associated with a lack of protein and other nutrients, from the present situation where micronutrients are supplied in adequate amounts. Life expectancy is increased if the number of calories taken a day is reduced by between 30 and 70 per cent, while still providing adequate amounts of essential nutrients. It appears that it is the number of calories that is important rather than the source of the calories. For example, it does not matter if the calories are reduced by removing fat or carbohydrate from the diet. In experiments with laboratory animals, giving vitamin supplements beyond those normally given does not increase life span.

In the present context the behaviour of the animals living on restricted diets is of interest. Most of us hope not for a long life, but for a long and vigorous life. The question has been examined in rats and mice. The behaviour of an old rodent fed a restricted diet has more in common with young animals than animals of the same age receiving more calories. Behaviourally there is no problem; the changes are for the better.

## Why does a low calorie intake increase life?

As restricting the diet so markedly decreases the rate of ageing, it is a phenomenon of great scientific interest. If we learn how a shortage of food alters our metabolism, then we may gain an important insight into the natural ageing process. We do not know why decreased food intake increases life span, although three mechanisms have been considered.[26]

Basal metabolic rate is the rate at which energy is expended by somebody who is fasting, resting and not using energy to maintain body temperature. Basal metabolic rate decreases as people get older, in part reflecting a decrease in the amount of muscle on the body. The eating of a low-calorie diet leads to a decreased metabolic rate. The first theory of why fewer calories in the diet increase the length of life is that it results in a reduction in the 'rate of living'. As the body lives at a slower rate, it can go on for longer.

In recent years there has been great interest in the possibility that much of the ageing process, and development of disorders such as cancer, may reflect the presence in the body of free radicals. Free radicals are chemically very reactive molecules that attempt to join themselves to other molecules to achieve a chemically more stable state. Once generated, free radicals promote the deleterious reactions that are the ageing process. Part of the interest in the anti-oxidant vitamins A, C and E, beta-carotene and selenium is their ability to increase the body's ability to mop up these free radicals.

The second theory of the way that a low-calorie diet may lengthen life is related to the first. It is suggested that as energy restriction reduces metabolic rate, there is reduced production of free radicals and hence damage to the cells.

Thirdly, changes in energy intake may influence the secretion of hormones. Homeostasis is the tendency for the body to keep various basic aspects of its physiology, such as blood glucose levels, within a prescribed range. There are many observations that suggest that ageing is associated with a general decrease in homeostatic capacity. The body is less able to rapidly achieve optimal internal states. Hormonal mechanisms play many roles in homeostatic mechanisms and the release of many hormones is influenced by a restricted calorie intake.[27] For example, a diet containing fewer calories decreases the release of adrenaline, which may be responsible for the lowered metabolic rate. One well-known feature of ageing is that the ability to control the level of blood glucose decreases. As we get older, after eating, blood glucose levels rise to higher values that fall more slowly. In animals a reduced-energy diet is associated with an increased ability to deal adequately with changes in blood glucose at an older age. The levels of blood glucose do not rise to such high levels and fall more rapidly.

## So you want to live to be 100?

The procedure that offers the most promise for a long life is the restriction of calorie consumption. Naturally it is a controversial topic, although two American researchers, Richard Weindruch and Roy Walford,[28] have suggested how you might proceed:

1 Calorie restriction should not be started before the age of 20, to allow growth to finish.

2 Calorie intake should be only gradually reduced until body-weight is 10 to 25 per cent below the stable weight without calorie restriction.

3 For males the intake is likely to be in the range 1,500–2,000 calories per day; for females, less.

Assuming that the procedure will work, you should think very seriously about the social and psychological implications of living many decades as an elderly person. Do you really want to live to 100? Do you really think that you can restrict your calorie intake for years on end? The generations of slimmers, whose weights have swung up and down throughout their lives, suggest that keeping weight at some prescribed low point is extremely difficult, if not impossible, for most people. To constantly keep body weight below its natural level will, for many, represent a severe decrease in their quality of life. Even if your life span is not extended, you may well have the impression that it has been.

If your aim is a vigorous, alert old age, then the restriction of calories brings with it many potential problems. The aim, remember, is 'undernutrition without malnutrition'. That's fine in principle, but not necessarily easy to achieve. Nutritionists often say that if you eat enough calories, then you need not worry about micronutrients, as they come associated with the calories. It follows that if you restrict calorie intake, there is a risk that you will become short of some vitamins, minerals or essential fatty acids. As we have seen, there is evidence that deficiencies of thiamine, folic acid and vitamin $B_{12}$ can result in neurological and psychiatric problems that vary from mild sensory and motor problems to overt psychotic behaviour. It would be advisable to talk to a dietitian to ensure that the new diet is not going to produce long-term problems.

After a review of the increasingly influential theory that ageing reflects the cumulative impact of the action of free radicals, an American researcher concluded:

It is reasonable to expect . . . that the healthy active life span can be increased 5 to 10 or more years by keeping body weight down, at a level compatible with a sense of well being, while ingesting diets adequate in essential nutrients but designed to minimize random free radical reaction in the body. Such diets would contain minimal amounts of components prone to enhance free radical reactions, e.g. copper and polyunsaturated lipids, and increased amounts of substances capable of decreasing free radical reactions, such as vitamin E, vitamin C, selenium, and the effective 'natural' anti-oxidants present in some foods, e.g. fruit and vegetables.[29]

This dietary recipe for a longer life has not been demonstrated to work; rather, it summarizes a large amount of current thinking. Although the ideas are derived from the study of ageing, they are familar. It is commonly suggested that if you keep your weight down, avoid fat and eat more fruit and vegetables, then you will decrease the likelihood of getting heart disease or cancer. It follows that you can expect to live longer.

It is important to place in perspective these dietary attempts to influence the ageing process so that false hopes are not generated. We are genetically programmed to age and eventually die. There is no evidence that we can extend the maximum age before which death must occur; the most we can hope to do is to make it more likely that we will get closer to that maximum age. The ageing process is inevitable.

# CHAPTER 11

# Diet and Mood

Of all the psychological changes that may occur when we eat, a change in mood is perhaps the one most commonly suggested. The effect may be general: for example, when we have eaten and drunk well, we experience a positive and relaxed view of the world. Alternatively, there have been repeated suggestions that specific nutrients have the ability to influence mood, in a similar way to a mild drug. In other cases a diet deficient in a particular mineral or vitamin may change your mood for the worse.

## *Do you use carbohydrate as a drug?*

Serotonin, or 5-hydroxytryptamine (5-HT), is one of the chemicals in the brain that pass messages from one nerve cell to another, a so-called neurotransmitter. The level of serotonin in the brain is known to be associated with mood, sleep, aggression, sexual behaviour and appetite. A major theory of the origin of depression is that it reflects a low level of brain serotonin. Many antidepressant drugs act by ensuring that the activity of brain serotonin is increased.

After we eat, protein is digested by the body and broken down into amino acids, the building blocks from which it is made. Tryptophan is one of about twenty amino acids that are commonly found in biological material. It is termed an essential amino acid: it cannot be manufactured by the human body, so it must be present in the diet. Tryptophan is important because it is converted into serotonin in the brain and influences our mood (Figure 11.1). What we eat

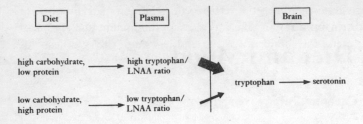

*Figure 11.1* **Conversion of dietary tryptophan into serotonin**
Tryptophan enters the brain by a mechanism that also transports five other large neutral amino acids (LNAA). Following a carbohydrate-rich meal, the relative concentration of tryptophan to the other LNAA increases: therefore more tryptophan enters the brain and is converted into serotonin.

in a meal influences the extent to which tryptophan enters the brain, but not in an obvious manner.

It might seem reasonable to suggest that if you ate a meal containing a high level of protein, there would be a higher level of tryptophan in the blood and that the rate at which it entered the brain would increase. The first part of the argument would be correct, but not the second. When you eat protein, the level of all amino acids in the blood rises, but, perversely, the amount of tryptophan entering the brain does not. Studies using laboratory rats have shown that it is a high-carbohydrate, rather than high-protein, meal that results in enhanced levels of serotonin synthesis in the brain.[1] Surely it should have been a high-protein meal that increased serotonin synthesis?

The answer to this puzzle was provided by Richard Wurtman at the Massachusetts Institute of Technology. Tryptophan enters the brain by a mechanism that also transports five other large neutral amino acids. Because the other neutral amino acids are present in protein in larger quantities than tryptophan, when you eat a high-protein meal, tryptophan is present in the blood to a relatively smaller extent. It follows that less tryptophan enters the brain. In contrast, when you eat a carbohydrate-rich meal, the associated release of insulin causes most amino acids to be removed from the bloodstream, but it has little effect on tryptophan. Following a carbohydrate-rich meal the relative concentration of tryptophan to the other neutral amino acids increases, so the amount of tryptophan that enters the brain increases and so does the synthesis of serotonin.

### Carbohydrate craving and depression

Depressive illness is a common psychiatric disorder that is characterized by a lack of interest and pleasure in everyday events, sleep disturbance, fatigue, poor concentration, feelings of worthlessness, and recurrent thoughts of death or suicide. Although there does not appear to be a single underlying social or biological mechanism that causes depression, a fall in the level of brain serotonin occurs in at least some cases. Drugs that deplete the brain of serotonin cause depression. Many antidepressant drugs increase the activity of serotonin in the brain. At post-mortem the levels of serotonin, its enzymes and breakdown products are lower in the brains of people who have committed suicide than in the brains of those who have died for other reasons. On the basis of evidence such as this a major theory of the biological basis of depression is that it reflects a deficiency of brain serotonin.[2]

In recent years an interest has developed in the relationship between appetite and depressive illness that owes much to the research of Richard and Judith Wurtman.[3] They suggest that when we eat carbohydrate, the level of serotonin in the brain rises. The increased level of serotonin changes our food preference: we no longer like carbohydrate to the same extent and eat other macronutrients. The Wurtmans have proposed that some obese people suffer from a disturbance of this feedback mechanism. When they eat a carbohydrate meal, the mechanism that stops further carbohydrate being eaten is not switched on. They therefore continue eating carbohydrate, whereas in others this desire would have been dampened by the increase in brain serotonin.

The Wurtmans used an interesting technique that gave obese patients access to a vending machine that provided a range of snacks. Some snacks were carbohydrate-rich and some were protein-rich. Every time a patient ate one of these snacks it was recorded by a computer. Unlimited quantities of food were supplied at mealtimes and the amount eaten was weighed.

It turned out that carbohydrate cravers do not eat more at mealtimes, but towards the late afternoon or early evening they begin to snack, almost entirely on high-carbohydrate foods. Almost half of the obese people who craved carbohydrate never took a protein snack, although they ate protein at mealtimes. The Wurtmans speculated that in these obese patients there was a malfunctioning of the mechanism in the brain that monitors carbohydrate intake.

When carbohydrate cravers were asked why they ate snacks, the response was rarely to do with hunger or the taste of food. Eating tended to make them feel clearheaded and calm. When they ate carbohydrate snacks were they attempting to manipulate their mood?

Judith Wurtman compared the reaction of people who craved carbohydrate and those who did not when given a carbohydrate-rich, protein-free meal. There was a different response. The carbohydrate cravers reported themselves as less depressed and more alert; the non-carbohydrate cravers felt sleepy and fatigued. It seemed to the Wurtmans that people eat carbohydrate snacks to improve their mood.

## Seasonal affective disorders

The winter and the darkness have slowly but steadily settled over us . . . The curtain of blackness which had fallen over the outer world of icy desolation has also descended upon the inner world of our souls . . . men are sitting about sad and dejected, lost in dreams of melancholy . . . For brief moments some try to break the spell by jokes, told perhaps for the fiftieth time. Others grind out a cheerful philosophy; but all efforts to infuse bright hopes fail.[4]

These comments from the journal of the Arctic explorer Frederick A. Cook, on 16 May 1898, describe winter depression. The long period of darkness in the Arctic winter had induced a depressive response. Today the disorder is called SAD, seasonal affective disorder, and occurs in susceptible individuals in the late autumn or early winter unless they move to latitudes where the day length does not decrease markedly at this time of the year. The symptoms can be controlled by simply sitting for several hours a day under bright artificial lights.

### Gill: a depressive who Craved carbohydrate

Gill was a teacher who every autumn felt tired and depressed. Every winter she put on weight and although only five foot two weighed over thirteen stone. She was only too aware that her weight problem resulted from eating carbohydrates. The stresses of teaching were such that in the afternoon she became anxious and tense, and ate carbohydrate to calm herself down. Her meals were largely pasta and bread. After school she kept nibbling food, in particular sweet things, until she went to bed. The behaviour varied with the time of year. It tended to start in the autumn, when she became barely capable of functioning either at school or at home. She started to crave carbohydrate and put on weight. In winter she slept for nine or ten hours a night, but still felt tired in the morning. In the spring she was a totally different person: full of energy, the craving for carbohydrate almost non-existent and most of the weight gained over the winter, lost. One winter a psychiatrist suggested that she should spend time each day sitting in front of a bright full-spectrum light. Within four days she was no longer depressed and the desire to eat carbohydrate had largely disappeared.

Recent interest in seasonal mood disorders was stimulated in the early 1980s when Peter Mueller, a psychiatrist at the National Institute of Mental Health in the United States, looked at the case of a 29-year-old woman whom he had been treating for winter depression. Over a period of years she had lived in several cities. Peter Mueller noted that when she lived further north, the depression started earlier in the year and lasted longer into the spring. When she had a winter holiday in Jamaica, her depression disappeared.

The obvious explanation was that it was the absence of sunlight that caused depression. He began to experiment with so-called photo-therapy, little more than sitting in front of a bright light. Within a week this patient's depression had disappeared.[5]

People with SAD typically eat more in the winter and put on weight. Some scientists say that the increased food intake reflects an attempt to decrease their depressive symptoms by eating carbohydrate-rich food.[6] In experiments it has been found that eating a carbohydrate-rich, protein-poor meal is associated with an improved mood in people with SAD.[7] The finding is consistent with the idea that high levels of carbohydrate lead to an increased synthesis of serotonin and hence to decreased depresssion.

## Carbohydrate craving and premenstrual tension

Premenstrual tension (PMT; also call premenstrual syndrome, or PMS) refers to negative changes experienced by some women, par-ticularly those in their 30s and 40s, just prior to the beginning of their menstrual period. The symptoms include water retention, irri-tability, anxiety, carbohydrate craving, sleep disturbance and lack of concentration. On occasions even suicidal and criminal behaviour have been related to the premenstrual stage.

A similar pattern has been observed in women who suffer with PMT and those with carbohydrate-craving depression and SAD. The Wurtmans examined women with PMT, and found that in the premenstrual period they, like some obese patients and those with SAD, increased their consumption of carbohydrate snacks, particularly chocolate. There was an association between changes in mood and eating carbohydrates: when the women became depressed they started to eat carbohydrates. Those women who did not report premenstrual symptoms did not increase their intake of carbohydrate snacks at this time.[8] Again, the Wurtmans suggested that the in-crease in carbohydrate intake is an attempt to increase serotonin synthesis and thus improve mood. Mood improved when a carbohydrate-rich, protein-poor meal was eaten by PMT sufferers in the premenstrual stage. When a similar meal was eaten at other stages of the menstrual cycle, or if it was eaten by women who stated that they did not experience premenstrual symptoms, the carbohydrate meal did not influence mood.[9]

When women were offered a series of foods at different stages of their menstrual cycle a clear pattern emerged. There was no significant difference in the amounts of ham, salted peanuts and salted snacks that were eaten, nor in the amount of bland foods eaten: unsalted peanuts, unsalted crackers, cheese. There was, however, a marked increase in the consumption of sweet foods – chocolate, coffee cake and gum drops – during the later stages of the menstrual cycle (Figure 11.2).[10] But was the increased food preference only for carbohydrate, or was it more general? When eight women recorded everything that they ate for sixty days, a characteristic pattern was observed (Figure 11.3). During the ten days prior to menstruation the percentage of calories consumed in the form of carbohydrates was greater than in the first ten days of the cycle. There was no significant difference in the intake of protein or fat

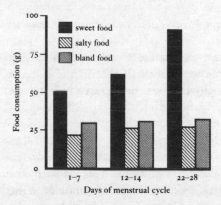

*Figure 11.2* **Food choice at different stages of the menstrual cycle**

Women were given a free choice of a range of foods, and the amount eaten at various stages in the menstrual cycle was calculated. Note that more sweet foods were eaten in the premenstrual stage.

*Source:* D. J. Bowen and N. E. Grunberg, *Physiology and Behavior*, 47, 1990, 287–91.

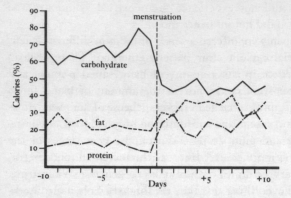

*Figure 11.3* **Carbohydrate intake at different stages of the menstrual cycle**

Everything that was eaten was recorded and the percentage of calories consumed in the form of carbohydrate, fat and protein was calculated. Note that in the ten days prior to menstruation there was a greater intake of carbohydrate.

*Source:* S. P. Dalvit-McPhillips, *Physiology and Behavior*, 31, 1983, 209–12.

throughout the cycle; however, the intake of carbohydrate during the first ten days of the cycle was only half that in the last ten days.[11] Again, it was as if carbohydrate was being eaten to influence mood.

## Sleep

Serotonin is important in the control of sleep. Animals with low levels of brain serotonin do not sleep; high levels of serotonin in the brain cause sleep. Thus if a high-carbohydrate meal increases the level of brain serotonin, it should be associated with feelings of sleepiness. After eating a high-carbohydrate meal females described themselves as sleepier and males described themselves as calmer.[12]

### Evaluation

The idea that people modify their food intake to modulate their mood is an intriguing one, but it is not without its problems. Although the evidence for such a mechanism exists, it is not the most robust phenomenon, and there is evidence that changes of serotonin levels in the gut, as well as in the brain, may play a part. More often than not the foods that are described as high-carbohydrate also contain large amounts of fat, for example chocolate and ice cream. So are the individuals concerned carbohydrate cravers, or are they fat cravers, or do they simply like the experience of eating pleasant-tasting foods? Not only do the high-carbohydrate foods contain high levels of carbohydrate and fat, but they often also contain some protein. In rats as little as 5 per cent of protein in a meal will suppress the ability of carbohydrate to enhance brain serotonin levels. If a similar mechanism also occurs in humans, then the ability of these craved foods to enhance brain serotonin levels must be seriously questioned.[13] It is highly unlikely that any high-carbohydrate meal would contain less than 5 per cent protein; alternatively, protein may still remain in the stomach from a previous meal.

These problems must lead us to question the idea that the consumption of high-carbohydrate foods can alter the level of serotonin in the human brain and hence modulate mood. In fact, the argument about changes in the level of brain serotonin relies on the extrapolation from rats to humans. If rats and humans turn out to be similar, it is improbable that serotonin synthesis will be influenced by diet. For brain serotonin to be influenced, we must eat a meal containing very little, if any, protein. With the exception of some drinks that are high in sugar, people rarely consume foods that are almost exclusively carbohydrate. However, even if high-carbohydrate meals do not influence serotonin levels in the human brain, it is well established that craving for carbohydrate occurs in some individuals, and that eating these foods is associated with improved mood.

## Low-fat diets and violence

The attempt to reduce cholesterol levels in the blood, by either the use of drugs or a low-fat diet, is one of the most widespread reasons for changing our diet. The hope is that we will decrease the chance of having a heart attack. In fact, there is an interesting suggestion that attempts to decrease blood cholesterol may increase the likelihood that we will have a violent death!

Cholesterol is an important part of all animal tissue, so some is present in all foods of animal origin, although some foods, such as egg yolks, have particularly high levels. Although it has had a bad press, cholesterol plays essential roles in the body: it is an essential part of cell membranes; it is the basic chemical from which a number of hormones are made; it is formed into bile acids. If you did not eat foods containing cholesterol, then the liver would have to make it.

You can, however, get too much of a good thing, and people with high levels of cholesterol in the blood are more likely to have heart disease. There is evidence that reducing blood cholesterol levels results in a lower incidence of death in people with a history of heart disease, and this has led to campaigns to persuade everyone to decrease the amount of fat they eat in the hope that it will decrease the rate of death from heart disease. Is there, however, evidence that a change in diet will benefit people without a history of heart disease?

When the medical profession wishes to establish that a procedure, such as a change in diet, influences the incidence of a particular disease, it has to monitor many thousands of people for many years. A group of researchers from the University of Pennsylvania have combined the data from six such trials, which have used drugs and changes in diet to reduce cholesterol.[14] As the results for drugs and diet are similar, they will be treated as one. The trials at which the researchers looked had all examined men aged 45 to 50 without a history of heart disease. Table 11.1 shows the main conclusions from a combined sample of nearly 25,000 men (12,457 who were, and 12,390 who were not attempting to reduce cholesterol levels) who were followed up for about five years. The attempts to

*Table 11.1* **Death rate in people using either drugs or diet to reduce cholesterol**

|  | Cholesterol reduction (%) | Control (%) | Significantly different |
|---|---|---|---|
| Total deaths | 4.74 | 4.50 | no |
| Death from heart disease | 1.36 | 1.59 | no |
| Death from cancer | 0.95 | 0.66 | yes |
| Death from causes other than illness | 0.53 | 0.30 | yes |

*Source:* Data from Muldoon *et al.*, *British Medical Journal*, 310, 1990, 309–14.

reduce cholesterol were successful: it was about 10 per cent lower in those who had attempted to reduce its levels. There was, however, no overall decrease in death rate: you were no less likely to die if you had changed your diet.

When specific reasons for death were examined, there were some surprising findings. Overall there was a trend for those who decreased their cholesterol levels to be less likely to die from heart disease, although according to normal statistical procedures the effect was not significant. More specifically, the use of drugs as opposed to diet to decrease cholesterol was more clearly associated with a decreased incidence of heart disease. A small increase in the rate of cancer occurred and remains a source of controversy.

Reducing cholesterol actually increased the incidence of death for reasons not related to illness. In fact, those whose cholesterol levels were lowered were more likely to have committed suicide, they were more likely to have had a road traffic accident and they were more likely to have been murdered!

Being murdered, killing yourself and having a car accident may at first sight have little in common. Was this an important observation or simply the product of unreliable data? The data seemed genuine. In the United States the rate of death from road accidents, murder and suicide is 62 per 100,000 of the population, for the age range of those in the six studies. In the control group, which had not attempted to reduce cholesterol levels, the rate was virtually identical, 64 per 100,000. There was every reason to think that they were typical members of society. In contrast the rate of death of those who had attempted to decrease their cholesterol was 107 per 100,000. The decreased likelihood of dying from heart disease was almost exactly matched by the increased likelihood of a violent death.

A possible explanation for these findings is that those who reduce their cholesterol levels are more aggressive. It is easy to see how those who are more aggressive will be more likely to have an accident while driving. It is a common suggestion that the motive behind suicide is self-directed aggression. Although murder by definition is committed by somebody else, it may be that somebody who is aggressive will be more likely to create a situation where somebody wishes to kill them. Support for this view came from monkeys fed a diet low in saturated fats and cholesterol, in fact a diet modelled on that recommended by the American Heart Association. If a monkey ate the low-fat diet, it was more aggressive than if it ate a diet high in fat and cholesterol.[15] Criminals with an antisocial personality, intermittent explosive disorder, aggressive conduct disorders or who are habitually violent when drunk tend to have low levels of cholesterol.[16]

The unexpected finding that decreasing cholesterol levels increased the likelihood of violent death led many researchers to look again at information they had collected to predict the incidence of heart disease. Initially, the findings were negative, those with low cholesterol levels were not significantly more likely to have committed suicide. The problem was that many studies had not examined a large enough group or had not carefully examined the nature of death or when it occurred. In Varmland, Sweden, over 25,000 men and 25,000 women had their cholesterol measured in the mid-1960s as part of a routine health check.[17] When the incidence of suicide was examined, the rate in men was four times greater if their cholesterol was in the lowest quarter rather than the highest quarter of the range (Figure 11.4). This association was not apparent in women, or in men more than six years after the level had been assessed.

If a low level of cholesterol was in part causing suicide, then an obvious prediction is that it will be associated with depression.

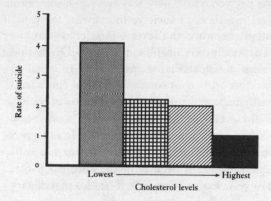

*Figure 11.4* **Cholesterol level and suicide**

The blood cholesterol level of 26,693 men was measured in 1964–5. The level of cholesterol was divided into quarters and related to the incidence of suicide in the next six years. The rate of suicide in men with the highest cholesterol levels was defined as one and other rates were compared with this. Note that those with the lowest cholesterol values were more than four times more likely to commit suicide.

*Source:* Data from Lindberg *et al.*, *British Medical Journal*, 305, 1992, 277–9.

An association between low cholesterol levels and depression has been reported on several[18] but not all occasions; age and other characteristics appear to be important in an as yet not totally clear manner.

How might changing the cholesterol levels in the diet influence the likelihood of suicide? Again, it has been suggested that serotonin might be involved.[19] In mice, when the level of cholesterol in the brain is increased, the number of sites at which serotonin acts also increases. When brain cholesterol levels decrease, the number of serotonin sites also decreases. As it is thought that serotonin suppresses aggressive behaviour and controls mood, this might account for the changes in behaviour.

Evaluation

Many of the associations between the level of cholesterol in the blood and suicide and depression are simply correlations. Depression is associated with a loss of appetite that might lead to a fall in cholesterol levels. Therefore we cannot conclude that low cholesterol causes depression; it may be that depression results in lower cholesterol. To distinguish these two explanations we need to decrease cholesterol levels while looking at the rate of suicide. Table 11.1 gives us the type of data we need. A decline in cholesterol levels was associated with increased suicide: such data allow the conclusion that changes in cholesterol levels change behaviour. The idea that dietary changes in cholesterol may have behavioural consequences is, however, so recent that it is fair to conclude that the jury is still out. Perhaps we should say, more accurately, evidence is still being collected.

A major function of cholesterol in the body is as a part of cell membranes. Although cholesterol as such does not enter the brain from the blood, fatty acids derived from diet do enter the brain and modify cell membranes.[20] Given the widespread campaigns to decrease plasma cholesterol levels by eating low-fat foods, it is surprising that the possible impact of such dietary changes on psychological functioning has attracted little attention. As about half the dry matter of the brain is fatty, it is reasonable to consider the possibility that change in the nature and amount of fat in the diet will have profound effects on brain functioning. The use of a high-fat diet to control epilepsy before the development of modern drugs showed that alteration in the fat content of the diet can influence brain functioning.[21] The association between low cholesterol levels and poor reaction times also supports the view that changes in diet may have psychological implications.[22]

These findings need to be kept in context. The effect on the rate of suicide was only apparent when tens of thousands of people were followed up. The increased rate of death due to suicide, murder and accident when cholesterol levels were decreased was only 0.2 per cent. It is not something for most of us to worry about. If you have a history of heart disease and are advised to consume a low-fat diet, then the advantages outweigh the disadvantages. Whether there is any point in people who do not have a high risk of heart disease

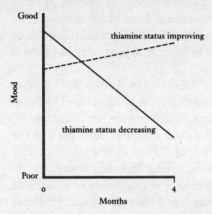

*Figure 11.5* **Thiamine status and mood**

Initially, those young adult females with poor thiamine status had a poorer mood; they were more likely to report feeling anxious or depressed. When given a vitamin supplement for four months, rising thiamine status was associated with better, and falling status with worse, mood.

*Source:* Adapted from Benton *et al.*, *Neuropsychobiology*, 32, 1995, 98–105.

attempting to decrease their fat intake is a question that is being debated increasingly in the medical literature.

## Vitamin status and mood

That low levels of vitamin $B_{12}$ and folic acid, and low thiamine status, may be associated with poor mood in elderly people was considered in Chapters 9 and 10. It appears that this association between vitamin status and mood may be true not only for the elderly. In a Welsh study of young healthy women there was an association between low thiamine status and feeling less composed, less confident and more depressed. When these women received vitamin supplements for three months, mood improved in those whose thiamine status increased (Figure 11.5). About 6 per cent of this Welsh sample of 20-year-olds had thiamine levels so low that mood was adversely affected.[23]

Similarly, in a large-scale German study the vitamin status of 1,228 young male adults was determined from blood samples. The 16 per cent with the poorest vitamin status were selected, and taking a vitamin supplement was found to improve mood (range of vitamins 2–4 × RDA).[24]

Thus there is increasing evidence from double-blind studies that there are sections of the population in industrialized societies whose mood would benefit from supplementation with vitamins or, better still, an improved diet. It should also be pointed out that the vitamin status of most of the population is sufficiently high that they do not benefit from supplementation. In the minority who do respond to vitamin supplementation it is reasonable to view these improvements in mood following supplementation with relatively low levels of vitamins as a response to a food supplement. The vitamins lacking from the diet have been supplied by taking a vitamin pill.

There is increasing interest in the possibility that taking vitamin supplements in excess of the RDA may decrease the incidence of cancer and cataracts.[25] The increasing tendency to recommend eating at least five or six portions of fruit and vegetables a day reflects, in part, an interest in the possibility that high doses of the antioxidant vitamins A, C and E decrease the incidence of various diseases. To date there has been only one similar study of the influence on psychological measures of high doses of vitamins for a long period.[26]

Young adults who took nine vitamins at ten times the US RDA for a year reported better mood. These improvements in mood occurred only after a year, although the levels of blood vitamins reached a plateau after three months (Figure 11.6). Clearly, such a profile cannot simply reflect the making good of a deficient diet; if this had been the case, then the improvement in mood would have been observed after three months. The improvement in mood was in particular associated with improved levels of riboflavin and vitamin $B_6$. The origin of this improved mood is uncertain, but the researchers speculated that it might reflect an increased production of serotonin in the brain. It is, however, difficult to come to any firm conclusion on the basis of a single isolated study. Certainly,

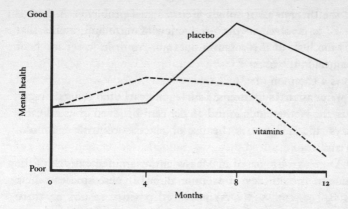

*Figure 11.6* **Influence of vitamin supplementation on mental health**

When young adult females took a multivitamin supplement for a year, towards the end they reported fewer symptoms of a minor psychiatric nature.

*Source:* Adapted from Benton *et al.*, *Neuropsychobiology*, 32, 1995, 98–105.

there was no suggestion that taking vitamin supplements had anything other than a small impact on mood. For the clinically depressed, vitamins are not an alternative to traditional drug or electro-convulsive therapy.

### Premenstrual symptoms

There is no generally accepted explanation of the origin of premenstrual symptoms. One theory is that it is associated with mechanisms that involve vitamin $B_6$. Vitamin $B_6$ plays an important role in the production of serotonin, dopamine and noradrenalin, three brain chemicals that all play important roles in passing messages from one nerve cell to another. As reductions in the neurotransmitters serotonin or noradrenalin are associated with depression, one theory is that the levels of these chemicals are lower in those suffering with premenstrual symptoms. Although often quoted as a justification for giving high doses of vitamin $B_6$, there is little hard evidence to support the theory that it solves premenstrual problems. Although vitamin $B_6$ is involved in the production of serotonin, a diet that provides too little of this vitamin does not result in lower levels of this chemical in the brain.[27]

It is a common idea that taking high doses of vitamin $B_6$ will relieve premenstrual symptoms: a survey of nearly 300 general practitioners in the Netherlands found 36 per cent believed in its efficacy. As always, the acid test is the use of placebo-controlled double-blind trials.

A Dutch group, based in Maastricht, examined a dozen of the best trials of the efficacy of vitamin $B_6$.[28] In these studies taking vitamin $B_6$ ($42-417 \times$ RDA) produced positive results on three occasions, negative findings on four occasions and in five studies the results were mixed. It is clear from these findings that the scientific evidence supporting the use of vitamin $B_6$ to relieve premenstrual symptoms is weak. All the studies to date have, however, used small numbers and there is a need for the topic to be examined on a larger scale.

There are several reasons why the scientific evidence and popular opinion on this topic may conflict. Firstly, the study of premenstrual symptoms is characterized by a beneficial response to a placebo in as many as 60 to 70 per cent of those studied. A large placebo response has a number of consequences. When vitamin $B_6$ is taken, a majority will respond positively because of the placebo response alone, giving the impression that it is a useful treatment. The question is whether there is in addition a pharmacological benefit. Even if there is a pharmacological benefit, it will be difficult to demonstrate when so many respond positively to a placebo. It is asking a great deal of any treatment that it will have such a dramatic impact that it is apparent in substantially more than 70 per cent of the population. This is a particular problem, as most studies make it clear that not all of those suffering with premenstrual syndrome benefit from vitamin $B_6$ supplementation. If there is only a subgroup of the population who benefit, then the improvement would be next to impossible to demonstrate in an unselected group. Yet how can we proceed when we have no means of selecting those who are likely to respond? Can we be sure that those who do not respond to vitamin $B_6$ are simply those who fail to produce a placebo response?

As vitamin $B_6$ is available without prescription, and it is very commonly promoted for the treatment of premenstrual symptoms, its use is likely to continue. It should be remembered that even if some women respond, there is no suggestion that all will. As there are fears that high doses of vitamin $B_6$ (over 500 mg) may cause damage to the nervous system, unsupervised self-medication of high doses is not recommended. Many doctors will be prepared to at least contemplate the use of this vitamin, although a range of other treatments should also be considered. The use of vitamin $B_6$ remains controversial.

Similarly, it has been postulated that when some women become depressed after starting to take the oral contraceptive, it may reflect a hormone-induced vitamin $B_6$ deficiency, which leads to a lower production of chemicals such as serotonin. The finding that the administration of vitamin $B_6$ (42 × RDA) decreased depression in those taking the oral contraceptive supports this view.[29] The status of this finding is again uncertain, as the topic has been the subject of little systematic examination.

## Minerals and mood

### Iron

Iron is the most abundant trace element in the body and, as it is distributed in an uneven manner, it is likely to perform different functions in various parts of the body. A shortage of iron is extremely common, particularly in women, resulting from the loss of blood during menstruation. Although iron shortage is a particular problem in non-industrialized countries, it is also a widespread problem in industrialized ones. A review of the topic concluded that 'iron deficiency and anaemia are the most prevalent nutritional disorders in the world. The behavioural changes induced by iron deficiency in adults include unusual lethargy, irritability, apathy, listlessness, fatigue, inability to concentrate, pica [appetite for, and eating, non-foods, such as soil and paint], inattention, hypoactivity and sometimes a decreased IQ level.'[30]

Iron is essential for the formation of haemoglobin, the chemical responsible for transporting oxygen around the body. If a body is not getting all the oxygen that it needs, a person will feel tired and depressed. Estimates suggest that about 20 per cent of the world's population is deficient in iron. If you are feeling abnormally tired, look for some of the tell-tale signs:

1 The inside of the eyelids are pale and colourless rather than pink.
2 The usual pinkness at the base of the fingernails has faded.
3 The lower lip and tongue are less pink than usual.
4 Physical effort is difficult to sustain and you become rapidly tired and lightheaded.

If you have reason to believe that you lack iron, then ask your doctor for a blood test, and if you are anaemic, iron supplements may be offered.

The body's reserves of iron are bound to the protein ferritin, the body's main store of iron. It is possible to have very low reserves of iron and not be anaemic. Thus the measurement of ferritin is a convenient and sensitive indicator of the early stages of iron deficiency.

There are high levels of iron in the brain. When the body is short of iron it is preferentially directed to the making of red blood cells. It is therefore possible that the levels of iron in the brain will become depleted although a person is not anaemic. If this occurs, then people without reserves of iron may have psychological problems. Joyce Fordy in Swansea surveyed young adults and used ferritin levels to distinguish those who had low iron reserves but were not anaemic.[31] Fifty-two per cent of females and 11 per cent of males had serum ferritin levels below the recommended level; that is, their iron intake was marginal. In males being vegetarian, and in females dieting, was associated with lower ferritin values. When a series of tests of psychological functioning was examined, marginal iron levels were associated with few psychological problems. There was, however, one exception.

Severe depression has been reported in about 6 per cent of women who use oral contraceptives, something that is true in only 1–2 per cent of women not using this form of contraception. In fact, depression is one of the most common reasons women stop taking the pill. Although it is commonly acknowledged that for a minority of women depression may be a side-effect of the use of oral contraceptives, the underlying reason is obscure.

The Swansea study of ferritin levels suggested a hypothesis: the oral contraceptive causes depression in women whose iron stores are depleted. In females taking the oral contraceptive, those with very low ferritin values were significantly more likely to report being depressed.[32] As always, such an observation needs to be interpreted cautiously, as it was only a correlation. Before concluding that low-iron status predisposes women to become depressed when they take the oral contraceptive, it must be shown in a double-blind trial that depression disappears when iron status improves. We await such data.

### Selenium

There are varying levels of the essential trace element selenium in soils throughout the world. As the level of soil selenium varies, so does the amount of selenium in the food chain, and hence in the human body. Plants do not need selenium, but the animals who live by eating the plants do. In areas such as New Zealand, the United Kingdom, and parts of China, Australia, Scandinavia and the United States the levels of selenium in food are so low as to suggest the possibility of deficiency, although to some extent the body may be able to adapt to a low intake. In a double-blind study carried out in Wales the taking of selenium (1.25 × RDA) was associated with a marked improvement in mood (Figure 11.7).[33]

Does this response to selenium suggest that the British diet supplies inadequate amounts of selenium? The evidence is limited, so, again, any conclusion should be cautious. Most selenium is consumed either in grain products or in meat. In 1978 the average British diet was calculated to provide approximately 60 $\mu$g of selenium per day.[34] More recently it was calculated that the intake of selenium had fallen to 43 $\mu$g a day,[35] as the wheat used for flour making was increasingly grown in the United Kingdom (on soil with low levels of selenium) rather than imported from Canada

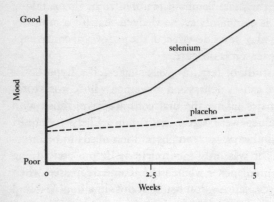

*Figure 11.7* **Influence of selenium supplementation on mood**

The taking of a selenium supplement for five weeks resulted in feeling less anxious, less depressed and more energetic.

*Source:* Data from Benton and Cook, *Biological Psychiatry*, 29, 1991, 1092–8.

(where soils have higher levels). The trend to eat less bread had also decreased the intake of selenium. The British figures recommend an intake of 75 μg a day for adult men and 60 μg a day for women, figures higher than those offered by many British diets. The origin of the improved mood following selenium supplementation is uncertain. Selenium is found in the brain and is concentrated in some areas rather than others, suggesting that it may play an important role in the brain's functioning that is as yet unsuspected. An important role for selenium in the manufacture of thyroxine by the thyroid gland has been discovered.[36]

Although an essential element, selenium is needed in very small amounts, and excess amounts are harmful. There is no suggestion that supplementation would be beneficial if the diet already provides adequate amounts. Anybody taking supplements should ensure that they do not exceed the recommended dose. It is likely that a response such as that in in Figure 11.6 will occur only in those parts of the world with low soil selenium. Again, there is no suggestion that a low intake of selenium is a cause of the psychiatric complaint of depression, and supplements do not offer an alternative to drug treatment.

## Final comment

Many aspects of diet have been associated with mood and mental health, including examples considered in other chapters. The amounts of the macronutrients fat, protein and carbohydrate have been implicated as well as various micronutrients. It may well be that mood is the psychological measure that is most sensitive to minor changes in diet. All nutrients serve a range of functions in the body and as such a deficiency may be expected to produce a range of often minor problems, at least in the first instance. Such minor problems may result in a person feeling slightly under the weather. It should not, however, be assumed that minor changes in the diet are the cause of, or the means of curing, major mood-related problems.

Perhaps the best way of looking at the association between diet and mood is to consider that a less than optimal diet will cause you to feel a little jaded. A diet that is right for you will result in you having fewer bad days. It should always be remembered that mood and mental health depend on many factors, and in most people diet is unlikely to predominate among them. There is, however, growing evidence that a poor diet may, to a limited extent, adversely influence mood.

# CHAPTER 12

# Meals and the Way You Think

Up to now much of the book has considered specific nutrients or foods, often in isolation from the rest of the diet. Clearly, we do not eat nutrients or foods in isolation; we consume meals that become our diet. This chapter considers meals, their common constituents and when they are eaten; and two drugs that we often consume with our meals, caffeine and alcohol.

## *Breakfast*

There is an aphorism that breakfast is the most important meal of the day, yet about a quarter of us choose not to eat breakfast, or at the most have a drink of tea or coffee. We have food in the kitchen, but we do not feel like eating first thing in the morning. If we eat our evening meal at six, miss breakfast and have lunch at one, then we have gone nineteen hours between meals. An obvious question is whether long periods between meals depletes the body of its energy reserves so that it is unable to perform efficiently. Are we psychologically more effective if we eat breakfast than if we miss it?

There have been relatively few attempts to assess the influence of eating breakfast, and evidence that it influences mood, attention and speed of reaction has not emerged. The strongest evidence is that the memory of people who do not eat breakfast is poorer late in the morning.[1] Figure 12.1 shows some of the results obtained by Pearl Parker in Swansea in a study in which memory was assessed in people who had and who had not eaten breakfast.[2] People who did not eat breakfast had poorer memory than people who did. However,

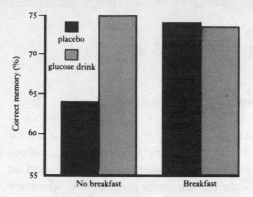

*Figure 12.1* **Breakfast and memory**
Subjects were asked to recall a list of three consonants (e.g., ZPK) after counting backwards for various periods of time. They received a glucose or artificially sweetened drink twenty minutes before testing began. If they had not eaten breakfast or had not consumed a glucose drink, then their memory was poorer.
*Source:* Adapted from Benton and Parker, *Journal of American Dietetics Association*, 1996, in press.

when people who did not eat breakfast drank a glucose drink, their memory was as good as those who had eaten breakfast. If a person eats breakfast, a glucose drink does not further improve memory.

Based on these and similar findings, it is tempting to suggest that fasting may deplete brain glucose to the extent that memory is disrupted. Although the poorer memory of people who have not eaten breakfast is a reason to recommend that a meal is taken first thing in the day, the findings should be kept in context. The improvement in performance is not general and appears to be most strongly associated with memory. The effects are observed when considerable demands are placed on the brain resources. There is only limited evidence that in everyday life a failure to eat breakfast is disruptive. Only where intense thought has been demanded throughout the morning is functioning likely to be sub-optimal. If you are taking a three-hour examination or your job demands that you pay attention to continuous incoming information, then eating breakfast may prove helpful.

## Lunch

When many real-life tasks are monitored throughout the day, a characteristic pattern emerges: performance decreases in the early afternoon. Figure 12.2 summarizes a few of these observations: train drivers are more likely to miss a warning signal, drivers are more likely to fall asleep and spinners work more slowly.[3] This decline has become known as the post-lunch dip in performance. There are two possibilities: firstly, that the decline in efficiency is a response to lunch and, secondly, that the decline reflects a bodily rhythm. The obvious way to distinguish these possibilities is to compare individuals who have and have not eaten lunch.

Initially, it appeared that the post-lunch dip was entirely a reflection of a bodily rhythm. A similar decline in performance was observed whether or not lunch had been eaten. More recently, this conclusion has been challenged. Professor Andrew Smith runs the Health Psychology Unit at the University of Bristol. He has found that some tasks are performed less well after eating lunch, whereas the performance of others is similar whether or not lunch has been eaten.[4] Tasks that are performed less well after lunch are those that require sustained attention. It now appears that the post-lunch dip reflects two underlying mechanisms. Firstly, there is a dip in our biological rhythm that results in decreased efficiency: we were meant to take a siesta. Secondly, eating lunch is associated with decreased efficiency, at least on tasks that demand our continued attention.

Eating larger rather than smaller lunches is associated with more lapses in attention in the early afternoon, although a drink containing caffeine will solve the problem.[5] Lunches high in carbohydrate result in reports of feeling lethargic and mentally slow.[6] People who consume a lunch with moderate levels of carbohydrate and fat rather than a meal with high levels of one of these macronutrients are more likely to describe themselves as cheerful and less

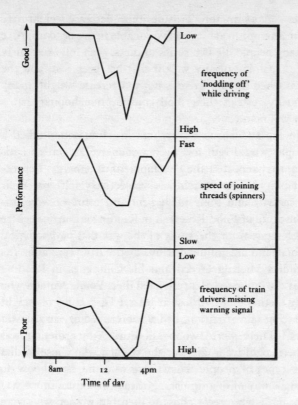

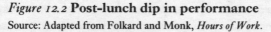

*Figure 12.2* **Post-lunch dip in performance**
Source: Adapted from Folkard and Monk, *Hours of Work*.

likely to describe themselves as drowsy and muddled.[7] The macro-nutrient content of lunch influences how people feel in the afternoon.

## Dieting

For many of us, much of the time, the problem is to decrease the size and frequency of meals. It has been estimated that at any one time one-third of the British population is dieting, something true of about 50 per cent of women. This desire to decrease weight may reflect either an attempt to achieve a fashionable figure or to improve health. For many people life is a series of diets, each followed fairly quickly by the regaining of any weight that has been lost, and the next diet. Even when the objective is not to decrease weight, many people continually restrict their food consumption hoping that a gain in weight will not occur.

When in the late 1940s researchers in Minnesota studied a group of people who lived for twenty-four weeks on a semi-starvation diet, they reported the development of lethargy, depression and irritability.[8] The individuals subjectively felt that their ability to concentrate and their judgement and memory were impaired. The Institute of Food Research in Reading is a major centre in the United Kingdom for the study of the way that psychological factors influence, and are influenced by, diet. Fifty years after the Minnesota studies Michael Green and his colleagues in Reading looked again at the influence of a restricted diet. Young women who were currently dieting and had lost at least 1 kg (2.2 lb) of weight were less able to sustain attention, had a poorer memory and slower reaction times.[9] There were two possibilities: either dieting was influencing their cognitive ability, or the women who chose to diet were different types of people from those who did not choose to diet. The obvious way of distinguishing these two explanations was to monitor not those who freely chose to diet, but women who were randomly asked to diet for the purpose of the experiment. Again, dieting influenced cognitive functioning; it was clear that it was the restriction of food consumption that was important. When the impact of missing one or two meals was examined, similar problems did not occur. These cognitive problems occurred only when food intake had been restricted for several days or weeks.[10] Similarly, problems in sustaining attention were found in people with the eating disorder *bulimia nervosa*, especially when there were biological signs of starvation.[11]

There are two explanations. As the dieters were consuming about 70 per cent of their normal diet, they may simply have been short of basic nutrients. Alternatively, it may be that the psychological effort of maintaining a diet uses up mental capacity that is not available for other activities.

## Food groups and psychological functioning

We all have an individual dietary style and prefer to eat certain types of food rather than others. When 7,076 British adults were asked how frequently they ate a list of foods, their responses fell naturally into obvious dietary categories.[12] For example, people who often ate one type of vegetable were more likely to eat other vegetables. People who ate one type of fruit or salad were more likely to eat similar types of food. A remarkable finding was associated with the eating of a group that was labelled fatty foods: crisps, chips, fried food, and sausage and meat products. There was an extremely strong association between eating these foods and the speed of reaction times (Figure 12.3): those who ate large amounts of fatty food had quicker reaction times, something true for both sexes, all ages and those from all social backgrounds. No similar association was found with other groups of food. The theory that intelligence is related to the speed of mental processing has attracted the attention of psychologists for many years. Reaction times are often used to measure the speed of mental processing. People with quicker reaction times score more highly in intelligence tests.

These types of finding are always difficult to interpret, as all we have is a correlation. Does a fatty diet increase reaction times or do people with quicker reaction times choose a particular diet? It is easy to suggest that eating fatty foods may be associated with a range of other characteristics, such as an increased likelihood to smoke, drink or avoid eating other kinds of food. As such, it is impossible to distinguish the influence of fatty foods from the associated lifestyle. Yet it is difficult to suggest an obvious aspect of lifestyle that would account for the findings. For example, eating fatty foods is associated with drinking alcohol. If alcohol consumption were the important factor, we would expect reaction times to be slower, not quicker. Although the label 'fatty foods' has been used, as there is no measure of fat intake, we cannot even be sure that fat intake is the important variable.

Is it reasonable to suggest that dietary fat influences brain functioning? A major function of cholesterol in the body is as part of cell membranes; in fact, lipids account for about half the dry matter

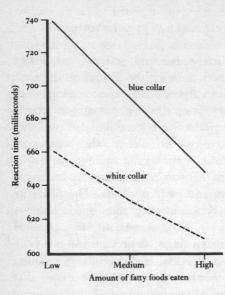

*Figure 12.3* **Association between eating fatty foods and reaction times**

A random sample of 7,076 British people was divided into thirds depending on the amount of fatty foods eaten. The reaction times of those eating higher amounts of fatty fats were quicker. This was true for all ages, both sexes and irrespective of whether they had white- or blue-collar jobs.

*Source:* Data from Benton, in Hillbrand and Spitz, *Lipids and Human Behavior*, 1996.

of the brain. It is, therefore, not unreasonable to suggest that anything that affects fat intake, and its metabolism in the body, may potentially influence the functioning of the brain. For example, before the development of anti-epileptic drugs, a high-fat diet was used to decrease the incidence of seizures. Even today it is suggested that a high-fat diet is helpful when drugs alone are unable to control seizures.[13] However, before we can conclude that the level of fat in the diet influences reaction times, it needs to be experimentally altered while any changes in reaction times are monitored.

A similar survey, carried out by Richard Cook in Swansea, related dietary style to mental health.[14] In women, but not men, there was an association between consuming large amounts of fruit and vegetables and being less depressed and anxious. Again, all of the problems of correlations occur with these findings. Does the diet improve mental health or do people with better mental health choose to eat in a particular way? In Chapter 11 and elsewhere the evidence that a low vitamin intake may be associated with poor mood was considered. It is possible that a better diet is associated with better mental health. Maybe the eating of large amounts of fruit and vegetables is associated with better micronutrient status, or perhaps some other constituent of diet is important. Given the evidence that a low vitamin intake occurs in only small sections of the population, this is not a likely explanation.

The relationship between mental health and fruit and vegetable consumption in females but not males suggests another explanation. Females are known to be more weight conscious, often limiting their food intake to prevent weight gain: fruit, vegetables and salad are frequently described as 'dieting foods', as they are low in calories. The possibility arises that those women who consume large amounts of fruit and vegetables are trying to enhance their self-image by maintaining a low body weight. Alternatively, those women with high self-esteem may be more inclined to slim and therefore tend to consume more fruit and vegetables. Thus good mental health may lead to the consumption of fruit and vegetables. Women with low self-esteem may be disinclined to watch their weight and therefore perceive no need to eat fruit and vegetables.

### Food craving

One factor that determines what we buy in a shop or choose from a menu are those foods that we feel an intense desire to consume. Food craving has usually been defined in a common-sense manner as the strong desire or urge for a particular food. The topic is of interest, as cravings are extremely common. Chocolate has been identified as by far the most craved food, to the extent that the

*Table 12.1* The frequency with which food is craved

| Food | Females (%) | Males (%) |
| --- | --- | --- |
| Chocolate | 39 | 14 |
| Pizza | 7 | 15 |
| Salty foods (crisps, popcorn, pretzels, salt) | 8 | 3 |
| Ice cream | 6 | 2 |
| Sweets and desserts | 6 | 4 |
| Meat and chicken | 3 | 5 |
| Bread and pasta | 3 | 2 |

One thousand Canadian students were asked which, if any, foods they craved. The data are reported as a percentage of the total who responded.

*Source:* H. P. Weingarten and D. Elston, *Appetite,* 17, 1991, 167–75.

terms 'chocolate addiction' and 'chocoholic' have been coined. When Harvey Weingarten asked 1,000 students at McMaster University in Canada, 97 per cent of women and 68 per cent of men reported experiencing cravings for food.[15] Table 12.1 lists the frequency with which particular foods were craved. Chocolate is in a class of its own; particularly for women, it is by far the most craved food item. It is apparent that food cravings are highly selective; relatively few foods are reported to induce cravings in other than a small minority of the population.

Eighty-five per cent of the Canadian students admitted that more often than not they gave in to their food cravings; clearly food cravings are powerful phenomena. Cravings do not seem necessarily to follow traditional food classifications. Usually, if people crave chocolate, only chocolate will satisfy that need; another sweet food will not fit the bill. If they crave potato crisps, another salty food will not be satisfying.

### Chocolate addiction?

Caviar is exquisite, but people don't declare their love with ten-pound heart-shaped boxes of it. Fresh figs are heavenly, but you don't find them on your hotel pillow at night. Entire magazines are not devoted to lobster or asparagus. But chocolate . . . chocolate inspires a passion normally reserved for things grander than food.[16]

Chocolate was introduced to Europe by early Spanish explorers, who discovered it in Mexico. The extent to which it has spread throughout the Old World and then back to the New is testimony to its great appeal. Without the availability of sugar to convert a basically bitter substance to a basically sweet taste, this could not have occurred.

The average person in the United Kingdom eats 9 kg (20 lb) of chocolate a year; on average, three bars a week.[17] In the United States the figure is 1.6 kg (3.5 lb) a year and in Switzerland 3.6 kg (8 lb).[18] In some people the consumption of chocolate is so great that analogies with drug and alcohol addiction have been drawn. When Marion Hetherington placed an advertisement in her local newspaper in Dundee, seventy-five people responded affirmatively to the question 'Are you a chocolate addict?'[19]

In fact, chocolate addiction is not a traditional psychiatric disorder, but it is clear that some people perceive it to be a problem. Many of the self-declared 'chocolate addicts' in Hetherington's study reported feeling stressed, lonely and depressed while craving chocolate. They experienced positive feelings while eating chocolate, although often this was followed by guilt. These chocoholics ate on average twelve and a half chocolate bars a week. One admitted to eating seventy bars a week – that's right, ten bars a day.

When 300 people answered 80 questions concerning chocolate, their responses fell into one of two groups.[20] Table 12.2 lists some of these questions. By far the most important dimension of the response to chocolate is whether you do or do not experience craving for chocolate. If the statements under the heading 'Craving' apply strongly to you, then you are a chocolate craver. The second way that we differ in our response to chocolate is the extent to which we

### Alice: a chocolate craver

Alice was 58 years old and lived alone. Throughout her life she had experienced chocolate craving and ate as much as 1 kg (2.2 lb) a day. She had no history of problems with eating disorders. Her mood had often been low, but when she had a major depression, she saw a psychiatrist. He treated her with an antidepressant drug. After about ten days her mood improved and for the first time in her life her craving for chocolate disappeared. Her appetite for other foods was normal; selectively, chocolate had lost its appeal. After six months her mood was normal and the chocolate craving had not reappeared. She had lost 9 kg (20 lb) in weight. Her psychiatrist noted that the loss of chocolate craving occurred before depression improved. Given that the antidepressant drug influences the brain's chemistry, he wondered if the chocolate craving had reflected some neurochemical abnormality.

---

feel guilty when we eat it. If the second series of comments applies strongly to you, then you feel guilty when you eat chocolate. These dimensions are independent. It is possible to experience intense chocolate craving and not feel guilty when you eat chocolate. Similarly, it is possible not to crave chocolate yet feel guilty when you eat it.

The lives of people who experience high levels of chocolate craving may be disrupted. The people who answered the questions referred to above tended to describe their craving as 'overpowering', said that they 'cannot get it out of their head' and that they 'cannot take it or leave it'. Chocolate was used at particular times: 'when I am bored', 'when I am upset', 'in the afternoon' and 'towards the end of the menstrual cycle'.

Scoring highly on the guilt dimension was not associated with eating a large amount of chocolate, and it may be that the guilt reflects a conflict between a high desire to eat chocolate and a self-imposed restriction. Those women who felt guilty were unhappy with their body shape and reported signs that may be indicative of

*Table 12.2* **Reactions to chocolate**

---

*Craving*

---

1  I eat chocolate to cheer me up when I am down.
2  My desire for chocolate often seems overpowering.
3  The thought of chocolate often distracts me from what I am doing.
4  I usually find myself wanting chocolate during the afternoon.
5  Even when I do not really want more chocolate, I will often carry on
eating it.

---

*Guilt*

---

1  I feel unattractive after I have eaten chocolate.
2  I feel guilty after eating chocolate.
3  If I resist the temptation to eat chocolate, I feel more in control of my
life.
4  I always look at the calorific value of a chocolate snack before I eat it.
5  After eating chocolate, I often wish I hadn't.

---

Reactions to chocolate fall into two groups: the experience of craving and guilt. If
the above comments apply strongly to you then you are high on the particular
dimension.

problem eating. They were more likely to report that 'I sometimes
force myself to be sick after eating chocolate'; 'I sometimes do not
eat chocolate for days and then eat a large amount in one go'; 'Even
when I do not really want any more chocolate I will often carry on
eating it.' A lack of control over eating, bingeing and self-induced
vomiting are behaviours that are typically associated with the eating
disorders anorexia nervosa and bulimia nervosa. It should be realized
that such comments were made only by people responding very
strongly to the types of questions in Table 12.2. A small amount of
guilt is very common and is not indicative of a problem.

Why is chocolate so attractive? Why is it so frequently craved?
Is this a drug-like response or a psychological reaction? Chocolate
certainly contains various substances that have pharmacological actions, including caffeine. A chocolate bar may contain 20 mg of
caffeine compared with 80–100 mg in a cup of coffee. This relatively

low dose and the fact that other sources of caffeine, such as coffee and cola drinks, are only infrequently craved, suggests that caffeine is not the major reason that chocolate is craved.[21]

Another substance in chocolate is phenylethylamine, which is also produced naturally by the body. In 1982 two New York psychoanalysts, Michael Liebowitz and Donald Klein, associated passionate love and chocolate. They found that a group of 'love-addicted' women whom they were treating produced a large amount of phenylethylamine. When the women's infatuations stopped, so did their production of phenylethylamine. As chocolate contains phenylethylamine, is chocolate a substitute for love?

Finally, chocolate contains very high levels of magnesium and it has been suggested that an attempt to increase magnesium intake may motivate the consumption of chocolate, particularly in the premenstrual period.[22]

To understand why people like chocolate we need to look no further than the sensory characteristics offered by chocolate. People who like chocolate tend to like other sweet-tasting items. Any sweet taste is innately attractive, and the combination of sweetness and high fat is particularly appealing. Chocolate melts at body temperature and produces a pleasing smooth texture in the mouth. It has a pleasant aroma. When these characteristics are reinforced, as they are in Western culture, by regarding chocolate as a luxury, which is given as a gift, often on special occasions to loved ones, it is not surprising that it is found to be so attractive.

## Alcohol

Alcohol, which is frequently consumed either by itself or with a meal, is a central nervous system depressant. Initially, it inhibits higher types of functioning, such as the ability to plan. Larger doses disturb perception and disrupt the control of the hands and legs. With still higher doses, memory is adversely affected and, finally, breathing and other basic biological mechanisms fail to function adequately. A safe conclusion is that any demanding task will be impaired after any amount of alcohol, however small.[23]

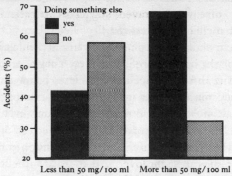

*Figure 12.4* **Blood alcohol levels and road traffic accidents**

People in road traffic accidents were asked whether they had been doing something other than driving immediately prior to the accident (e.g. lighting a cigarette). Those with higher levels of blood alcohol were more likely to have been doing something other than driving.

*Source:* Data from Brewer and Sandow, *Ergonomics*, 23, 1980, 185–90.

For one year a research team went to road traffic accidents in Adelaide, South Australia.[24] They obtained estimates of blood alcohol levels and interviewed the drivers. Their hypothesis was that people with alcohol in their blood would be less able to deal with a situation that demanded that their attention was divided. Figure 12.4 shows the findings. Those drivers who had blood alcohol levels above 50 mg per 100 ml were more likely to have been doing something other than simply concentrating on driving: lighting a cigarette, tuning the radio or trying to get something out of their pocket. The higher levels of alcohol may have influenced the situation in various ways. Those with higher levels of alcohol may have been less likely to inhibit a tendency to do something other than driving, or when faced with two tasks, they may have been less able to deal with the additional demands.

Although the law of many countries sets a level of blood alcohol above which it is illegal to drive, the evidence is that even levels below the limit decrease efficiency. The impact of a small dose of alcohol is similar to that which occurs with fatigue, boredom and many commonly prescribed drugs. Small doses of alcohol are not uniquely a problem nor necessarily a major problem: hence the level of blood alcohol at which you can legally drive is set above zero. The legal limit for driving in Britain is blood alcohol level below 80 mg per 100 ml, although in some countries it is 100 mg per 100 ml.

In the short term alcohol acts as a relaxant and may even improve performance that has been disrupted by anxiety or stress. It is the most commonly used anti-anxiety drug. The disinhibiting effect of alcohol can result in people speaking more freely than usual without the worry of the long-term consequences of their behaviour.

People often attempt to limit alcohol consumption when some demanding activity, such as driving, is anticipated. To do this, they need to judge their degree of intoxication. People who are asked to estimate their degree of intoxication, judge that it reaches its peak sooner than in fact it does. After a single drink, blood alcohol level peaks nearly half an hour after people subjectively feel that it has. Alcohol-induced disruption of functioning peaks when the blood alcohol level reaches its maximum, and not at the earlier point when people think that it has. People also tend to overestimate the rate at which intoxication decreases. The difference between a subjective estimate of being sober and a measure of blood alcohol level can vary by two hours.[25] These observations show that self-assessment is an unreliable means of judging when you are fit to drive. If you believe, in error, that your alcohol level has already peaked, then you might drive while the level is still increasing.

Men and women metabolize alcohol differently. The blood alcohol level tends to peak sooner in women, and sooner and at a higher level in the premenstrual stage of the menstrual cycle. It is well established that if a person eats prior to drinking alcohol, then the blood alcohol level does not reach the same height. Although alcohol still disrupts performance, it does so to a smaller extent when a person has eaten.[26]

Drinking alcohol leaves people with a hangover. Many of us will view a hangover as the headache and other symptoms that remain the morning following the night before. When these physical symptoms have disappeared, or even if they never existed, there may be a hangover in the sense that psychologically people are not at their most efficient: 'Drinking also leaves a residual impairment on sober performance for at least fourteen hours and plausibly much longer after large doses.'[27]

The morning following a heavy drinking bout it is possible that the level of blood alcohol is still sufficiently high that it would be illegal to drive. Even if the legal level has been achieved, psychological efficiency will be below normal and a person would be well advised to avoid driving. When pilots were tested in a flight simulator, their performance was significantly worse fourteen hours after drinking moderately (blood alcohol levels 100 mg per 100 ml) than when they had abstained.[28] Their subjective rating of their performance on the simulator did not differ, however: they were unaware that their performance was impaired.

## Caffeine

For many people the final stage of a good meal is a cup of coffee. The start to a good day is that first cup of tea or coffee. Consuming drinks containing caffeine is probably the most common attempt to use diet to alter psychological functioning. Caffeine occurs naturally in a number of foods and is added to others for its drug-like properties. The vast majority of the population will drink coffee or a similar substance to fight sleepiness, maintain alertness or counteract the influence of alcohol.

Table 12.3 lists the dose of caffeine present in a range of common drinks and other products. If you note the number of caffeine-containing substances you consume a day and refer to Table 12.3 you will be able to estimate your caffeine intake. In 1978 in the United States the daily consumption of caffeine was estimated to be 29 mg a day in children aged 2–5 years, 43 mg a day in children aged 6–17 and 186 mg a day in people 18 and older.[29] These data may not reflect the high levels of caffeine consumed by those children who drink large amounts of cola drinks. In the United Kingdom it has been estimated that the average adult caffeine intake is 444 mg a day, reflecting the relatively high consumption of tea and coffee.[30]

*Table 12.3* **Availability of caffeine**

| | |
|---|---|
| Brewed coffee | 85 mg/150 ml |
| Instant coffee | 60 mg/150 ml |
| Decaffeinated coffee | 3 mg/150 ml |
| Brewed tea | 50 mg/150 ml |
| Instant tea | 30 mg/150 ml |
| Cocoa | 6–142 mg/150 ml |
| Cola drinks | 32–65 mg/150 ml |
| Aspirin/caffeine products | 30–65 mg/tablet |
| Pep pills | 100–200 mg/tablet |

The principal action of caffeine is to stimulate the central nervous system, but it also increases the production of urine, stimulates the heart and relaxes smooth muscle. Very high doses of caffeine release adrenaline, which produces physiological changes similar to those associated with anxiety or stress.

Reaction times are frequently used as a measure of how quickly the brain can process information. It has been consistently reported that doses of caffeine over 200 mg a day produce quicker reaction times, although with lower doses the findings are equivocal. Doses in excess of 100 mg a day improve the ability to sustain attention.[31] There is very little evidence that caffeine, at any dose, influences learning and memory. Doses of caffeine of 100 mg or more a day increase reports of alertness and decrease reports of fatigue. However, doses in excess of 400 mg a day are more likely to result in feelings of anxiety. Students who consumed over five cups of coffee a day have been found to be more anxious and depressed.[32]

There is agreement that taking caffeine is associated with a postponement of going to sleep. A dose of 100 mg or greater half an hour prior to going to bed postpones sleep. However, doses of 80 mg or less have not produced detectable changes.[33] While caffeine has been consistently found to influence sleep, there are individual differences and its effect is highly dependent on the pre-existing level of fatigue or boredom. Caffeine in doses from 300 to 500 mg has been found to increase the capacity to do physical work.[34]

### Are we all addicted to caffeine?

There is little doubt that it is possible to become addicted to caffeine. As with all drug addiction, withdrawal symptoms occur when administration of the drug is stopped. The case study of Nigel gives one such example. Headaches and feelings of tiredness are the most commonly reported withdrawal symptoms, while anxiety, craving, nausea, vomiting and impaired psychomotor performance are mentioned less frequently. Withdrawal symptoms have been documented after the consumption of 600 mg a day for only 6–15 days. The withdrawal syndrome has an onset 12–24 hours after the last intake and lasts for about a week.

---

### *Nigel: a caffeine addict*

Nigel worked as a computer programer, and had recently taken a new job. Although during the week he felt normal, every weekend he felt low. He had headaches and nausea, he was tired and anxious. Strangely, although he left for work on Monday morning with the symptoms, they soon disappeared, only to reappear the following Saturday morning. His moods at the weekend placed a strain on his relationship with his wife, Heather, who associated his bad temper with spending time with her. Only many months after starting work in the new office was a solution suggested by a friend, who wondered if the problem was not what he did at the weekend but rather what he did in the week.

The office had a constant supply of strong, filtered coffee; it was the job of one of the secretaries to ensure that it never ran out. Nigel drank one mug of coffee after another. Any office meeting or talks with a client always started with coffee. Nigel estimated that he drank at least six mugs of coffee a day at work and others with breakfast and after an evening meal. Colleagues thought this an underestimate. A friend who had visited him at work suggested that Nigel's problems might result from an addiction to caffeine and that every weekend he was displaying withdrawal symptoms. Nigel felt this was unlikely but, to please his wife, agreed to stop drinking coffee in the office for a trial period. On the Monday in

question he felt worse than he usually did at weekends: he felt
stiff, had a severe headache and actually vomited. The symptoms
improved over a period of about a week and did not reappear.
Nigel was convinced that his problem was caffeine addiction and
from that time stopped drinking drinks containing caffeine. He
now feels well at the weekends and his relationship with Heather
has much improved.

---

When a person takes a drug regularly, it is common for tolerance to occur: the body adapts by changing its basic biochemistry so
that the drug has less impact. When tolerance has occurred, more
drug is needed to achieve the same effect as the initial dose. Tolerance occurs with caffeine: a dose that would initially have influenced
a person psychologically, with repeated use no longer has the same
impact. The dose needs to be increased to obtain a similar effect.

As most people consume less than 600 mg of caffeine a day,
the question arises as to whether lower doses of caffeine are similarly
addictive. In a very careful study carried out in the Johns Hopkins
University in Baltimore, Maryland, the answer was yes.[35] People
consuming caffeine equivalent to two and half cups of coffee a day,
about 235 mg, were given either a placebo or their usual amount of
caffeine in a capsule, so that they were unaware what they were
taking. When they received the dummy tablets for two days – that
is, they no longer had caffeine in their diet – they showed withdrawal
symptoms. They reported themselves as more depressed, anxious
and tired. Fifty-two per cent reported moderate headaches or headaches so severe that they took aspirin. The conclusion must be that
the majority of people in Western societies are addicted to caffeine
to the extent that if they stop consuming it they will display withdrawal symptoms.

Withdrawal symptoms will be most noticeable if consumption
of the substance is abruptly stopped. People who want to decrease
their caffeine intake may wish to do so gradually over several weeks
and thus avoid the more severe problems. The withdrawal of caffeine
has been recommended as part of the treatment of anxiety and
symptoms such as awareness of palpitations, which are rapid heart-
beats, and insomnia.[36]

*Figure 12.5* **Caffeine**

---

1 Caffeine acts on the brain to increase alertness and help sustain performance.

2 The doses required to produce these effects will occur only if a person drinks several strong mugs of coffee very rapidly.

3 A single high dose or a high cumulative intake can produce anxiety-like symptoms.

4 For most people consuming drinks containing caffeine does little more than prevent withdrawal symptoms. Withdrawal symptoms occur when caffeine is removed from the diet.

---

### Children's reactions

The possibility that the repeated consumption of caffeine may adversely influence children's development has been a matter of concern, although the basis of the concern is unclear, as there has been little research. Normal boys given either 100 or 369 mg of caffeine a day have been reported to be more active, have faster reaction times and better attention.[37] There is, however, little evidence of a response to the amount of caffeine likely to be consumed when drinking normal quantities of soft drinks.

An insight into the possible impact of repeatedly consuming caffeine comes from clinical studies in which caffeine is administered for medicinal purposes to infants who spontaneously stop breathing. When a large dose of caffeine (20 mg/kg) was administered from birth to two years, bodily growth and neurological and psychological development were found to be normal.[38] In these cases the dose of caffeine was several times that which could be consumed by dietary means. Thus, although giving caffeine to growing children has sometimes been a cause of parental worry, there is little hard experimental evidence to justify these concerns.

# CHAPTER 13

# What Should You Do About Your Diet?

There are various ways that diet has been said to influence behaviour:

1 Low blood glucose levels can produce psychological disruption.

2 Food intolerance causes behavioural problems.

3 Inadequate intakes of vitamins and minerals cause characteristic problems.

4 Differences in our basic biology mean that some of us require 'mega' doses of vitamins.

Conventional medical opinion is that all these suggestions should be treated largely, if not totally, with contempt. If these phenomena occur at all, they do so infrequently. For most of the population they are irrelevant. The book has summarized some of the evidence supporting the view that any generalization that diet never causes psychological problems is too strong a statement. Certainly, for the first three items on the list there is good evidence that at least some of us are influenced psychologically by our diet. That megavitamins may be helpful, in anyone other than rare individuals, is much less certain.

What should we do about our diet if we wish to be at our peak psychologically? One of the messages of this book is that we are all individuals, and our lifestyle and basic biological make-up will influence our dietary needs. To the extent that needs are individual, meaningful general advice cannot be offered. This final chapter, however, suggests some general principles that may prove helpful.

## Low blood glucose

Hypoglycemia, frequently diagnosed and rarely confirmed, remains in the public view; some authors consider it the cause of symptoms ordinarily associated with anxiety as well as a factor in violent crime and automobile accidents . . . We find misdiagnosis of hypoglycemia potentially harmful. It can delay the detection of serious problems.[1]

Indeed, although diet can induce the very low level of blood glucose that is needed for a clinical diagnosis of hypoglycaemia, it is a rare phenomenon, not a problem for the vast majority of the population (see Chapter 7). In drawing this conclusion it should not be assumed that food-induced falls in blood glucose are never a problem. For people with this predisposition, it can have serious consequences. However, a related but more minor phenomenon does appear to be of more widespread concern.

Although the blood glucose level does not influence mood and psychological efficiency in many circumstances, it can be important when people are faced with long-term and intense demands. In part our biological nature is important. Some people are better able to transport glucose to the brain rapidly when the need arises. How recently they have eaten is also critical: we have seen that drinks containing glucose improve the memory of people who had not had breakfast (Chapter 12).

The solution to both food-induced hypoglycaemia, on the rare occasions that it occurs, and a decline in psychological efficiency over time is the same. Eat regularly; do not miss meals; eat more small meals rather than a few large ones.

## Food intolerance

When the Royal College of Physicians reviewed the area of food intolerance, it said:

Irritability and depression are among the symptoms which may accompany food intolerance, but it remains to be established whether foods can provoke psychiatric problems alone, unaccompanied by other symptoms which would suggest a tissue reaction elsewhere . . . There are also claims that hyperactivity in children can be improved by dietary manipulation, including avoidance of additives, but this has been the subject of considerable controversy.[2]

It seems that such a conclusion is too strong. The use of a double-blind approach in cases such as Joanna's (see Chapter 5) allows us to be certain that for some people food intolerance can be the cause of psychiatric problems. If the authors of the report are asking whether food intolerance influences the brain directly, rather than there being a psychological reaction to the disrupted functioning of some other area of the body, this is an academic point. By whatever means it occurs, people such as Joanna clearly respond to their diet with serious psychiatric symptoms. Since this report was written well-designed studies have shown that for some, but not all, hyperactive children food intolerance is the cause of their behavioural problems (see Chapter 6).

It should not be assumed that food intolerance is anything other than an unusual problem. Few adults who display psychiatric symptoms or children who become hyperactive are responding to their diet. The probability is that when a serious behavioural problem is considered, it is not food-induced. If it is food-induced, then there are dozens of food items that may potentially play a role. Only a long systematic examination of the diet will reveal which foods are a problem in each case.

## Subclinical deficiencies of vitamins and minerals

In Chapter 1 we saw that a vitamin deficiency disease is extremely unlikely, but that subclinical deficiencies – those not severe enough to produce a deficiency disease – can have psychological consequences. There is an increasing number of scientific studies that have found that aspects of the psychological functioning of apparently healthy members of industrialized societies have benefited from vitamin supplements. We have seen, for example, that taking micronutrients can improve mood (Chapters 9, 10 and 11), memory and attention (Chapter 9) and intelligence scores (Chapter 4). Typically, not everybody responds, but rather a minority distinguished as having a poor vitamin or mineral status. These responses to supplementation have been found in double-blind placebo-controlled studies, and therefore are difficult to dismiss.

### Vitamin intake and psychological functioning

Many of the ways that a low vitamin intake can influence bodily functioning are summarized in Figure 13.1. As the body's reserves of a particular vitamin decrease, the activity of enzymes that require that vitamin also decreases. Enzymes are proteins that drive chemical reactions in the body. Such a decline in biochemical efficiency is often the first physiological sign of a suboptimal vitamin intake. In fact, the activity of enzymes in red blood cells is used to establish whether somebody has an adequate store of various B vitamins.

If the deficiency persists, the disturbance becomes more severe: a so-called deficiency disease results and will eventually damage the body. However, in the case of some vitamins the first signs of a marginal vitamin intake, a long time before a deficiency disease is apparent, are psychological. For example, depression,

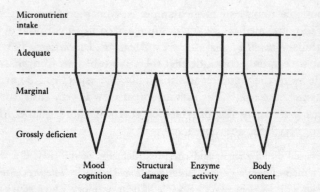

*Figure 13.1* **Micronutrient content and bodily functioning**

hysteria and hypochondria appear earlier than the symptoms of an outright deficiency disease when there is an underconsumption of thiamine, riboflavin, niacin and vitamin C. Marginal intakes of vitamin $B_{12}$ and folic acid can result in depression and dementia in the elderly, as we saw in Chapter 10.

The above comments are non-controversial. What is less certain is the frequency with which the psychological symptoms associated with a marginal intake of a vitamin occur in industrialized societies. Indeed, whether psychological problems are commonly caused by marginal vitamin intake is the subject of great controversy. It appears unlikely to many nutritionists that in such societies the intake of micronutrients will be even marginally deficient. The argument is that the diet supplies sufficient protein and calories, and the necessary micronutrients come associated with them. However, we have seen that nutritional surveys, rather than finding that diet is universally good, point to sections of the population with a marginal intake (Chapter 2). With thiamine in particular there seems to be good evidence that the psychological functioning of a section of the population is disrupted by a marginal intake (see Chapter 9).

## Megavitamins

The possible impact of megavitamins is even more controversial. The traditional medical view was summarized in an editorial of the prestigious *Journal of the American Medical Association*: 'For the present we can only conclude that there is no benefit from massive daily doses of the vitamins and that only one aspect can be evaluated, namely the risk.'[3] The establishment view is very clear: megavitamins are largely the province of charlatans and quacks. The taking of very large doses of vitamins is:

largely based on an ancient and cherished delusion of the laity: if a small dose of a medicament is good, a larger dose may be better. The procedure is in conflict with an elementary principle of pharmacology which states that increasing the dosage of a therapeutic compound leads to maximum effectiveness and, on further increase, to the production of toxic effects.[4]

*Figure 13.2* **Advice about vitamin–mineral supplements**

---

1 Only in extreme cases will you benefit from taking vitamin–mineral supplements. There is much more to diet than vitamins and minerals, and it is better that these micronutrients are consumed as part of an otherwise adequate diet.

2 Eat a varied diet; take more of your calories in the form of unrefined carbohydrate rather than sugar and fat; ensure an intake of five or more portions of fruit and vegetables a day.

3 If you believe that your diet is inadequate and you are not prepared to change it, you may wish to take a vitamin–mineral supplement as an insurance policy. As long as you are aware that it is possible that you are wasting your money, then that is your decision.

4 Nutritional surveys have found that people taking supplements in most cases have a better diet without the supplements than people who do not take supplements. In other words the section of the population that takes supplements includes those people least likely to benefit from them.

---

Although there is truth in many of the details of these statements, do they tell the whole story? The pharmacological principle that beyond a certain level any additional micronutrient will do no good, and may do some harm, is well established. What the comment misses is the basic premise of those people who suggest that in exceptional cases very large doses may be beneficial. Their argument is that some of us need vast doses of micronutrients, presumably in most cases for genetic reasons. Such people simply lack the ability to efficiently move micronutrients to those areas of the body where they are needed.

There is no disputing that an excess of a vitamin will do you no good: an excess is, by definition, more than is needed. The real question is whether the need for a vitamin or mineral can differ markedly. Do some people require an intake vastly greater than others, and if they do not obtain these large doses, do psychological symptoms result?

## *Are you an average or an individual?*

Medicine has progressed by the study of average rather than individual responses, and for many purposes this has proved very successful. Medical textbooks make statements that are 'true' for everybody, yet whenever we examine any human characteristic we find natural variation. We are all very similar, but we are not identical.

When a doctor takes a sample of blood or other bodily tissue and measures something in the laboratory, the results are related to a normal range. If the measure is between A and B, then the level is acceptable; if it is outside this range then the reading is abnormal. Depending on the measure, the difference between A and B may be relatively large. Although people are similar in their make-up, they are not identical.

As an analogy, let us consider the height of the human male. The genetic background of the race of which a man is a member will be important; the average height of men from different racial backgrounds will differ. If we consider only caucasian men from northern Europe, there is still a substantial range of heights. Exceptionally, perfectly normal males may reach a height of 2.08 m (6 ft 10 in) or more. Perfectly normal males may also be about 1.52 m (5 ft) in height. Most of this male population is between 1.67 m (5 ft 6 in) and 1.82 m (6 ft). In a situation where height is important, for example the design of a car seat, we can do little but deal with these average figures. We may design a seating position that would suit men between 1.67 m (5 ft 6 in) and 1.82 m (6 ft), and it will prove acceptable for the vast majority of men in this particular population. However, for men at either the lower or higher end of the normal range of height, the seat will prove to be uncomfortable or even dangerous.

The view that some people have a genetically determined need for a high intake of a micronutrient is called the genetotrophic approach. It can be seen in a similar manner to height and the design of car seats. Statements about nutritional needs are usually based on average responses. There is no incompatibility between the suggestion that most people in the population receive adequate levels of vitamins and minerals and the suggestion that some people need much more than an average intake. If your genetics dictate that you need much more than the average intake of micronutrients, is there any reason to view you as more unusual than somebody who is 2 m (6 ft 6 in) tall? We gain a great deal of understanding by viewing people as individuals and not assuming that everyone has similar needs and responds to a given situation in a similar way.

Roger Williams, who directed the Biochemical Institute of the University of Texas, devoted a major portion of his career to the development of the concept of biochemical individuality. In his view, emphasizing the ways in which people differ from each other adds to our understanding of medical disorders. He drew together basic information from many areas of human biology, pointing out how much people can differ.[5] One area he considered was nutritional need.

For example, when calcium intake is studied in the laboratory, the amount needed to maintain bodily levels can vary by as much as 400 per cent. When nine volunteers were fed the same diet, designed to offer inadequate levels of thiamine, four developed symptoms of the deficiency disorder beri-beri, one was borderline and four displayed no symptoms. The important point is that there are substantial differences in the ability to function on a given intake of a nutrient.

Similarly, when individuals live in a situation where the diet offers a marginal intake of a particular nutrient, some develop deficiency diseases, and some do not. One example Williams uses was the occurrence of scurvy on sailing ships before the need to offer citrus fruit as a source of vitamin C was appreciated. In a crew eating the same diet one crew member might have died of scurvy, whereas others had mild symptoms and some were completely symptom free. Later, laboratory studies showed that the amount of vitamin C needed to saturate the body could differ four-fold from person to person.

Another example concerned areas, for example parts of England and Switzerland, where locally grown food offered iodine in amounts smaller than those required. In groups eating the same diet some adults developed the deficiency disorder goitre and some young children developed the physical and mental problems known as cretinism. However, many people in these areas did not develop these deficiency diseases.

A third example focused on parts of the United States where in the early decades of this century the diet of poor people offered too little niacin. Again, whereas some people developed the deficiency disorder pellagra, most did not. It is difficult to escape the conclusion that people can differ quite markedly in the level of nutrients they require to prevent the development of deficiency symptoms.

The data collated by Roger Williams support the view that some people require a higher intake of particular nutrients. If it is accepted that the first signs of a minor nutritional deficiency are, in many cases, psychological, then we would predict that the psychological functioning of a minority would benefit from a change in diet. Whether there is a nutritional equivalent of somebody who is 2.08 m (6 ft 10 in) is less certain. This analogy would suggest that there are a few people in the population who need many times the average intake to satisfy their genetically determined abnormally high nutritional needs. As Vincent Marks suggested, these people might need to see a doctor. It may well be that their unusually high needs reflect the inability of their body to absorb, metabolize and store the nutrient in a normal manner. Such an analysis suggests that we should expect such individuals to respond to high doses of vitamins. The hard-nosed scientist might accept the argument that such a position is possible, but will demand evidence that it is in fact the case. In such an area evidence is difficult to obtain. The double-blind approach will make sense only if all the members of the group examined have the same problem. If we wanted a large group of people over 2.08 m (6 ft 10 in) in height we would have difficulty in finding them, even though height is immediately obvious. If we want a group of people who need very high doses of a vitamin, there is no obvious way of finding them.

Realistically, we are left with studies of individuals. In Chapter 1 Clare's need for a higher than normal intake of chromium was described.[6] In this case the use of a double-blind approach means that we can be certain that her persistent headaches reflected a need for chromium in higher doses than her diet offered. Her diet offered chromium at a level equivalent to the British RDA, but she required more. Such cases, although rare, strongly support the genetotrophic approach. There is no obvious answer to the question 'How do I know if I need a high level of a nutrient?'

## What should you do about your diet?

Having very nearly finished reading this book, and having had described a series of situations in which at least some people have benefited from a change in diet, what should you do? How can you tell if your diet is adequate? Can you be sure that your problems do not reflect your diet?

There are no easy answers. There is no straightforward way of establishing whether you do or do not eat a diet that is adequate for you. However, an impression that has repeatedly arisen is that where a response to diet has been demonstrated, it has arisen in a minority of the population. For example, although there are several reports that vitamin supplementation improves mood, this has happened only in cases where those with the lowest levels of vitamin have been studied. It seems that if you consume a good diet, you are unlikely to have a problem; but what is a good diet?

### A good diet

Throughout the Western world governments have been recommending changes in diet to reduce disease and improve health. Although these recommendations differ in detail, they have much in common:[7]

    1 Reduce fat consumption, in particular saturated fat.
    2 Decrease consumption of sugar and alcohol.
    3 Increase the consumption of dietary fibre.
    4 Eat a varied diet.
    5 Maintain a desirable body weight.

More specific suggestions are that you should eat five or more servings of fruit and vegetables a day. This will supply

*Figure 13.3* **Dietary advice for optimal psychological functioning**

---

1 Eat regular meals. Small meals eaten regularly will keep you psychologically more efficient than one or two large meals a day.

2 Eat breakfast: low blood sugar later in the morning adversely influences memory. Similarly, a mid-afternoon snack will help to keep you going when you begin to flag.

3 Decrease the amount of saturated fat and sugar in the diet, and replace the calories with unrefined carbohydrate. Eat five or six servings of fruit and vegetables a day, which will offer both fibre and vitamins and minerals. Eat plenty of wholemeal bread, pasta and brown rice.

4 Be sure you consume enough iron, particularly if you are female. Liver and red meat offer excellent sources. Wholegrain cereals, pulses and green vegetables also offer iron, although less is absorbed by the body. A drink containing vitamin C, such as orange juice, will aid absorption of iron.

5 Include oily fish, such as herring, sardine, mackerel and salmon, in your diet. They offer a good source of essential fatty acids, which play important roles in the brain. Pregnant and lactating women in particular should ensure that they have sufficient essential fatty acids, as these are important for the developing brain of foetus and child.

---

dietary fibre, vitamins and minerals, and may also offer various substances that are being examined for their possible anti-cancer properties. There is also reasonable evidence that decreasing dietary levels of saturated fatty acids can reduce the incidence of heart disease.

While the major aim of the nutrition message of the health education lobby is to reduce the incidence of heart disease, cancer, stroke, diabetes and bowel problems, similar dietary advice can be offered for its psychological benefits (see Figure 13.3). If you eat such a diet you should not need to take supplements. To be sure you are getting the full range of vitamins and minerals, look at Table 13.1 and ensure that you eat a varied diet.

*Table 13.1* **Sources of vitamins and minerals**

| Vitamins | |
|---|---|
| Biotin | Liver, kidney, egg yolk, milk, wholegrain cereals |
| Folic acid | Liver, green vegetables, wholegrain cereals |
| Niacin | Meat, liver, fish, nuts, wholegrain cereals, milk and dairy products, eggs |
| Pantothenic acid | Liver, kidney, eggs, milk, wholegrain cereals |
| Riboflavin | Meat, milk and dairy products, eggs, fish, pulses (beans, peas, lentils), fortified breakfast cereals |
| Thiamine | Bread, grain products, fortified breakfast cereals, meats, pulses |
| Vitamin A | Liver, oily fish, margarine, milk, meat, carrots, green vegetables |
| Vitamin $B_6$ | Meat, milk, wholegrain cereals, potatoes, pulses, eggs, vegetables |
| Vitamin $B_{12}$ | Meat, fish, eggs, milk, cheese |
| Vitamin C | Fruit and vegetables, citrus fruit, green vegetables, potatoes |
| Vitamin D | Oily fish, margarine, butter, eggs |
| Vitamin E | Vegetable oils, green vegetables, eggs, wholegrain cereals |
| Vitamin K | Green leafy vegetables |

| Minerals | |
|---|---|
| Calcium | Milk, dairy products, bread, green vegetables |
| Copper | Wholegrain cereals, meat, vegetables |
| Iodine | Meat, milk, eggs, fish |
| Iron | Liver, red meat, wholegrain cereals, pulses, green vegetables |
| Magnesium | Bread, cereals, potatoes, milk, vegetables |
| Selenium | Meat, cereals, milk, eggs |
| Zinc | Meat, bread, wholegrain cereals, milk |

# Glossary

**Acetylcholine** a neurotransmitter (passes messages between nerve cells).

**Adrenaline** a hormone produced by the adrenal glands and released during stress and when blood glucose is low.

**Alzheimer's disease** disorder of ageing characterized by loss of memory and inability to form new memories.

**Amino acids** the building blocks from which protein is made.

**Anaemia** lack of red blood cells.

**Anorexia** loss of appetite.

**Anorexia nervosa** psychiatric disorder where there is fear of putting on weight, an obsession with thinness, to the extent that death due to starvation may occur.

**Antigen** usually a protein but sometimes a polysaccharide that the body recognizes as foreign, and which is capable of provoking an immune response.

**Beta–carotene** found associated with chlorophyll, the pigment that in plants is necessary for photosynthesis; can be converted into vitamin A.

**Bulimia nervosa** an eating disorder characterized by a tendency to binge and then induce vomiting or use laxatives to prevent weight gain.

**Calcium** mineral essential for bone, teeth and brain functioning.

**Carbohydrate** general term for sugars, starches and cellulose.

**Cellulose** one of the main constituents of dietary fibre.

**Cholesterol** fatty substance with essential functions in body: insulates nerve cells; building block from which hormones are made; formed into bile acids. Found in food of animal origin.

**Choline**   water-soluble member of vitamin B complex; not a true vitamin, as it can be synthesized in liver.

**Clinical deficiency**   an intake of a micronutrient so low that a deficiency disease occurs.

**Complex sugar**   disaccharide.

**Decilitre**   tenth of a litre.

**Deficiency disorder**   a physical disorder caused by a lack of a particular vitamin, e.g., beri-beri and pellagra.

**Diabetes mellitus**   disorder in which blood glucose is high because the pancreas fails to release insulin.

**Dietary reference values**   a term used instead of RDA in the most recent British assessment of dietary needs.

**Disaccharide**   a sugar consisting of two linked monosaccharides, e.g., sucrose formed from glucose and fructose.

**Dopamine**   a neurotransmitter (passes messages between nerve cells).

**Double-blind**   a trial where neither the patient nor the doctor knows who is receiving a placebo or active treatment.

**DRV**   dietary reference values.

**E102**   tartrazine, a yellow–orange food dye.

**Eczema**   red, itching, scaling of skin.

**Elimination diet**   diet that contains only a few foods that are unlikely to induce food intolerance.

**Enzyme**   a protein that drives a chemical reaction in the body.

**Essential amino acid**   one that cannot be made by the body, and therefore must be part of the diet.

**Essential fatty acid**   one that cannot be made by the body, and therefore must be part of the diet.

**Fat**   a macronutrient that consists mainly of a mixture of triglycerides.

**Fat-soluble vitamin**   vitamins found in dietary fat; does not dissolve in water. Vitamins were originally thought to be either fat soluble (A) or water soluble (B). It is now known that there are several fat-soluble vitamins: A, D, E and K. *See also* water-soluble vitamin.

**Fatty acid**   fat consists of a mixture of triglycerides, which, in turn, consist of combinations of three fatty acids and glycerol.

**Ferritin**  protein that stores iron.

**Fibre**  the indigestible parts of food; roughage; e.g., cellulose, lignins and pectins.

**Folic acid**  water-soluble vitamin, member of vitamin B complex.

**Food allergy**  a response to food involving the immune system.

**Food aversion**  an adverse psychological reaction to food.

**Food-induced hypoglycaemia**  low blood glucose stimulated by food.

**Food intolerance**  a general term for the many biological ways in which the body may be unable to deal adequately with food.

**Genetotrophic**  the view that some people have a genetically determined need for a high intake of a micronutrient.

**Glucagon**  hormone produced by the pancreas that causes the liver to release glucose.

**Glucocorticoids**  hormones released by the adrenal glands in response to stress; involved in glucose metabolism.

**Glucose Tolerance Test**  test of ability to control blood glucose by monitoring changes after the consumption of a drink containing glucose.

**Haemoglobin**  the iron-containing molecule in red blood cells that binds oxygen.

**Hippocampus**  area of the brain thought to be important in memory.

**Histamine**  chemical released from mast cells as part of an allergic reaction.

**5HT**  5-hydroxytryptamine: *see* serotonin.

**Hyperactivity**  excessive activity.

**Hypoglycaemia**  abnormally low levels of glucose in the blood.

**IgE**  Immunoglobulin E.

**Immune response**  reaction to antigen by antibody production.

**Immune system**  defence mechanism against bacterial and viral infection.

**Immunoglobulin** (Ig)  family of proteins from which antibodies are derived. There are five main classes. Immunoglobulin E (IgE) is most closely associated with immediate allergic responses.

**Immunological**  concerned with immunity.

**Insulin**  hormone released by the pancreas that is responsible for the movement of glucose from the blood into the cells.

**Iron**  essential trace element needed to produce red blood cells; a deficiency of iron in the diet results in anaemia.

**Korsakoff's syndrome**  a disorder in which brain damage is associated with problems of memory; a shortage of dietary thiamine is a common cause.

**Lactose**  milk sugar, a mixture of glucose and galactose.

**Lecithin**  mixture of choline, fatty acids and other substances.

**Linoleic fatty acid**  essential fatty acid.

**Lipids**  general term for all fatty substances.

**Macronutrient**  general term for fat, carbohydrate and protein.

**Meal Tolerance Test**  a means of testing the ability to control blood glucose in which glucose is administered with fat and protein.

**Megavitamin therapy**  treating a disorder with doses of vitamins above those found in even a good diet.

**Microgram ($\mu$g)**  one-thousandth of a milligram.

**Micronutrient**  vitamins and minerals; nutrients required in small amounts.

**Milligram**  one-thousandth of a gram.

**Mineral**  Literally means mined from the earth; divided into metallic elements, such as calcium and magnesium, and non-metallic elements, such as sulphur, iodine and selenium.

**Monosaccharide**  simple sugar such as glucose or fructose.

**Neural tube**  spinal column.

**Neurone**  the basic cell of the nervous system; passes electrical messages.

**Neurosis**  group of psychiatric disorders characterized by unrealistic anxiety.

**Neurotransmitter**  chemical that passes messages from one nerve cell to the next.

**Noradrenaline**  a neurotransmitter (passes messages between nerve cells).

**Niacin**  water-soluble vitamin of B complex.

**Nicotinamide**  active form of niacin.

**Nicotinic acid**  active form of niacin.

**Oedema**  Swelling of body due to retention of fluid.

**Oligoantigenic diet**    a diet of a few foods all of which are unlikely to cause problems of food intolerance.

**Orthomolecular approach**    an attempt to achieve the level of micronutrients in the body that allows optimal functioning.

**Pancreas**    gland that releases insulin and glucagon.

**Phenylalanine**    An amino acid.

**Phenylketonuria**    a genetic disorder in which the amino acid phenylalanine is not correctly broken down; if untreated, associated with intellectual impairment.

**PKU**    phenylketonuria.

**Placebo**    a dummy treatment with which an active treatment is compared.

**Placebo response**    getting better for psychological rather than physiological reasons.

**Polyunsaturated fatty acids**    (PUFA) tends to be applied to linoleic, linolenic and arachidonic acids.

**Post-lunch dip**    a decrease in psychological efficiency that occurs in the early afternoon.

**Protein**    essential nutrient that is digested to produce amino acids, which are absorbed and rebuilt by the body into its own proteins.

**Psychosomatic**    a bodily change that originates in the mind.

**Psychosis**    a serious psychiatric disorder, such as schizophrenia or depression, where the person is out of touch with reality.

**Pyridoxine**    vitamin $B_6$.

**RDA**    recommended daily allowance (USA), recommended daily amount (UK).

**Reactive hypoglycaemia**    low blood glucose that is a reaction to food.

**Recommended daily allowance/amount**    daily minimum requirement of vitamins and minerals that will prevent deficiency disease in 95 per cent of the population.

**Riboflavin**    vitamin $B_2$.

**Salicylates**    chemicals that are similar to salicylic acid, aspirin.

**Saturated fat**    Fat with no double bonds in its molecules, making it stable; most animal fats are saturated.

**Saturated fatty acid**    Fatty acid with no double bonds in its molecules, making it stable.

**Scurvy** deficiency disorder caused by lack of vitamin C.

**Selenium** essential trace element.

**Serotonin** biologically active chemical found in brain, gut and blood platelets, and thought to be important in the control of mood; also known as 5-hydroxytryptamine (5-HT).

**Simple sugar** monosaccharide.

**Single blind** study where the patient does not know if a placebo or active treatment is being given but the doctor does.

**Spina bifida** disorder of development where spinal column does not completely encase the spinal cord.

**Spontaneous hypoglycaemia** another name for food-induced hypoglycaemia.

**Starch** a long chain of units of glucose.

**Subclinical deficiency** minor problem caused by a low intake of a micronutrient not sufficient to produce deficiency disease.

**Sucrase** enzyme that breaks down sucrose.

**Sucrose** a disaccharide, a combination of glucose and fructose; the sugar most commonly added to food.

**Sugar** colloquial name for sucrose, in plural used as general term for all mono- and disaccharides.

**Tartrazine** E102 a yellow–orange food dye.

**Thiamine** vitamin $B_1$.

**Trace element** elements that are needed by the body in small amounts.

**Triglyceride** a molecule containing glycerol and three fatty acids; fat in foods consists of a mixture of triglycerides.

**Tryptophan** amino acid that in the brain is converted to the neurotransmitter serotonin.

**Tyramine** an amine sometimes found in food that can cause a rise in blood pressure; normally destroyed rapidly by liver.

**Unsaturated fat** fat with double bonds in its molecules, making it chemically reactive; all fish oils and most vegetable oils (except coconut and palm) are unsaturated.

**Vitamins** essential components of diet required in small quantities that cannot be made by the body. When supplied in too small amounts a characteristic deficiency disease results, which can be cured only by a supply of the particular vitamin.

**Vitamin A**    fat-soluble vitamin known as retinol.

**Vitamin B$_1$**    water-soluble vitamin; thiamine.

**Vitamin B$_2$**    water-soluble vitamin; riboflavin.

**Vitamin B$_6$**    water-soluble vitamin; pyridoxine.

**Vitamin C**    water-soluble vitamin; ascorbic acid.

**Vitamin D**    fat-soluble vitamin, occurs naturally as cholecalci-ferol (D$_3$) in foods of animal origin; substantial amounts produced by action of sunlight on skin.

**Vitamin E**    fat-soluble vitamin known as alpha tocopherol.

**Water-soluble vitamin**    vitamin found dissolved in water; some B vitamins and vitamin C are water soluble; *see also* fat-soluble vitamin.

**Wernicke's Syndrome**    disorder characterized by memory problems; caused by a lack of thiamine.

**Zinc**    essential trace element.

# References

## 1. Are You What You Eat?

1 R. Mackarness, *Not All in the Mind*, London, Pan Books, 1976.
2 C. Fredericks and H. Goodman, *Low Blood Sugar and You*, New York, Constellation International, 1969, p. 2.
3 H. Tryphonas, 'Factors possibly implicated in hyperactivity', in R. L. Trites (ed.), *Hyperactivity in Childhood*, University Park Press, 1979, p. 93.
4 F. Prince and H. Prince, *Feed Your Kids a Better I.Q.*, Slough, Middlesex, W. Foulsham & Co, 1987.
5 A. Hoffer, M. Walker and R. J. Williams, *Nutrients to Age without Senility*, New Canaan, Conn., Keats Publishing, 1980.
6 H. B. Van Dyke, 'The weapons of panacea', *Scientific Monthly*, 64, 1947, 322.
7 A. K. Shapiro, 'A contribution to a history of the placebo effect', *Behavioral Science*, 5, 1960, 109–35.
8 Council on Food and Nutrition, 'Vitamin preparations as dietary supplements and as therapeutic agents', *Journal of the American Medical Association*, 1, 1959, 41.
9 *Independent*, 2 Oct. 1990.
10 J. H. Kellogg, *The Itinerary of Breakfast*, New York, Funk and Wagnalls, 1919.
11 J. T. Dwyer, W. H. Dietz, G. Hass and R. Suskind, 'Risk of nutritional rickets among vegetarian children', *American Journal of Diseases of Children*, 133, 1979, 134–40.
12 R. E. Olsen, 'Vitamin $B_{12}$ deficiency in the breast-fed infant of a strict vegetarian', *Nutrition Review*, 37, 1979, 142–4.
13 R. Cook and D. Benton, 'Chromium supplementation improves chronic headaches: a case study', *Journal of Nutritional Medicine*, 3, 1992, 61–4.

## 2. What's Important in Your Diet?

1 Food and Nutrition Board Subcommittee on the Tenth Edition of the RDAs, *Recommended Dietary Allowances*, Washington, DC, National Academy Press, 1989, p. 1.

2 Panel on Dietary Reference Values of the Committee on Medical Aspects of Food Policy, *Dietary Reference Values for Food Energy and Nutrients for the United Kingdom*, London, HMSO, 1991, p. 2.

3 R. J. Williams, *Biochemical Individuality*, New York, John Wiley and Sons, 1956.

4 D. Benton, 'Vitamin–mineral supplements and intelligence', *Proceedings of the Nutrition Society*, 51, 1992, 295–302.

5 J. Garrow, 'New Dietary Reference Values', *British Medical Journal*, 303, 1991, 148.

6 Panel on Dietary Reference Values, *Dietary Reference Values*, p. 5.

7 Department of Health and Human Services, *The Surgeon General's Report on Nutrition and Health*, Washington, DC, US Government Printing Office, 1988.

8 J. M. D. Malvy, M. S. Mourey, C. Carlier, P. Caces, L. Dostalova, B. Montagnon and O. Amedee-Manesme, 'Retinol, B-Carotene and a-Tocopherol status in a French population of healthy children', *International Journal of Vitamin and Nutrition Research*, 59, 1989, 29–34.

9 Quoted in G. Cannon, *The Politics of Food*, London, Century, 1987.

10 ibid.

11 *Daily Telegraph*, 3 Apr. 1986.

12 Subcommittee on Nutritional Surveillance; Committee on Medical Aspects of Food Policy, *The Diets of British Schoolchildren*, London, HMSO, 1989.

13 'The Threatened Generation', Granada Television, 14 April 1986.

14 ibid.

15 *Daily Telegraph*, 2 Feb. 1988.

16 ibid.

## 3. Early Influences

1 J. Ortega Torres, 'Effects of malnutrition in pregnancy and childhood on early brain development: methodological, pathophysiological, anthropological and psychological considerations', *Journal of Clinical Nutrition and Gastroenterology*, 3, 1988, 69–80.

2 J. Dobbing, 'Infant nutrition and later achievement', *Nutrition Reviews*, 42, 1984, 1–7.

3 R. M. Garfield and P. F. Rodriguez, 'Health and health services in Central America', *Journal of American Medical Association*, 254, 1985, 936–43.

4 D. E. Barrett and D. A. Frank, *The Effects of Undernutrition on Children's Behavior*, New York, Gordon and Beech, 1987, pp. 162–3.

5 A. Chavez and C. Martinez, *Growing Up in a Developing Country*, Mexico City, Instituto Nacional de Nutricion, 1982.

6 D. P. Waber, L. Vuori-Christiansen, N. Ortiz, *et al.*, 'Nutritional supplementation, maternal education and cognitive development of infants at risk of malnutrition', *American Journal of Clinical Nutrition*, 34, 1981, 807–13.

7 S. K. Joos, E. Pollitt, W. H. Mueller and D. L. Albright, 'The Bacon Chow study: maternal nutritional supplementation and infant behavioral development', *Child Development*, 54, 1983, 669–76.

8 Barrett and Frank, *Effects of Undernutrition*, pp. 189–90.

9 Waber *et al.*, *American Journal of Clinical Nutrition*, 34, 1981, 807–13.

10 W. R. Beardslee, P. H. Wolff, I. Hurwitz, R. Pankh and H. Shwachman, 'The effects of infantile malnutrition on behavioral development: A follow-up study', *American Journal of Clinical Nutrition*, 35, 1982, 437–41.

11 E. S. Susser, P. II. Shang and P. Lin, 'Schizophrenia after prenatal exposure to the Dutch Hunger Winter of 1944–1945', *Archives of General Psychiatry*, 49, 1992, 983–8; Z. Stein, M. Susser, G. Saenger and F. Marolla, 'Nutrition and mental performance', *Science*, 178, 1972, 708–13.

12 Stein *et al.*, *Science*, 178, 1972, 708–13.

13 D. Rush, Z. Stein and M. Susser, 'A randomized controlled trial of prenatal nutritional supplementation in New York City', *Pediatrics*, 65, 1980, 683–97.

14 L. E. Hicks, R. A. Langham and J. Takenaka, 'Cognitive and health measures following early nutritional supplementation: a sibling study', *American Journal of Public Health*, 72, 1982, 1110–18.

15 A. Lucas, R. Morley, T. J. Cole *et al.*, 'Early diet in preterm babies and development status at 18 months', *Lancet*, 335, 1990, 1477–81.

16 M. H. Poole, B. M. Hamil, T. B. Cooley and I. B. Macey, 'Stabilization effect of increased vitamin $B_1$ intake on growth and nutrition of infants: basic study', *American Journal of Disorders of Children*, 54, 1937, 726–49.

17 R. F. Harrell, E. R. Woodyard and A. I. Gates, 'The influence of vitamin supplementation of the diets of pregnant and lactating women on the intelligence of their offspring', *Metabolism*, V, 1956, 555–62.

18 R. W. Smithells, S. Shephard, C. J. Schorah *et al.*, 'Possible prevention of neural-tube defects by periconceptional vitamin supplementation', *Lancet*, i, 1980, 339–40.

19 MRC Vitamin Study Research Group, 'Prevention of neural tube defects: results of the Medical Research Council vitamin study', *Lancet* 338, 1991, 131–7.

20 J. B. Dunn and M. P. M. Richards, 'Observations on the developing relationship between mother and baby in the neonatal period', in H. R. Schaffer (ed.), *Studies in Mother–Infant Interaction*, New York, Academic Press, 1977.

21 H. B. Young, A. E. Buckley, B. Hamza and C. Mandarano, 'Milk and lactation: some social and developmental correlates among 1000 infants', *Pediatrics*, 69, 1982, 570–84.

22 A. Lucas, R. Morley, T. J. Cole, G. Lister and C. Leeson-Payne, 'Breast milk and subsequent intelligence quotient in children born pre-term', *Lancet*, 339, 1992, 261–4.

23 R. Morley, R. Cole, R. Powell and A. Lucas, 'Mother's choice to provide breast milk and developmental outcome', *Archives of Disease in Childhood*, 63, 1988, 1382–5.

24 M. Makrides, M. Neuman, K. Simmer *et al.*, 'Are long-chain polyunsaturated fatty acids essential nutrients in infancy?', *Lancet*, 345, 1995, 1463–8.

25 E. M. Widdowson, 'Mental contentment and physical growth', *Lancet*, i, 1951, 1316–18.

## 4. Intellectual Growth

1 J. R. Flynn, 'Massive IQ gains in 14 nations: what IQ tests really measure', *Psychological Bulletin*, 101, 1984, 171–91.

2 R. Lynn, 'The role of nutrition in secular increases in intelligence', *Personality and Individual Differences*, 11, 1990, 272–85.

3 D. Benton and G. Roberts, 'Effect of vitamin and mineral supplementation on intelligence of a sample of schoolchildren', *Lancet*, i, 1988, 140–43.

4 S. J. Schoenthaler, S. P. Amos, W. E. Doraz, M. A. Kelly and J. Wakefield, 'Controlled trial of vitamin–mineral supplementation on intelligence and brain function', *Personality and Individual Differences*, 12, 1991, 343–50.

5 M. Nelson, D. J. Naismith, V. Burley, S. Gatenby and N. Geddes,

'Nutrient intakes: vitamin–mineral supplementation in British school-children', *British Journal of Nutrition*, 64, 1990, 13–22.

6 L. W. Po, 'Vitamins, IQ and the Law', *Pharmaceutical Journal*, 1992, 506–8.

7 I. K. Crombie, J. Todman, G. McNeill *et al.*, 'Effect of vitamin and mineral supplementation on verbal and non-verbal reasoning of school-children', *Lancet*, 335, 1990, 744–7.

8 D. Benton and J-P. Buts, 'Vitamin–mineral supplementation and intelligence', *Lancet*, 335, 1990, 1158–60.

9 I. K. Crombie, J. Todman, G. McNeill and C. du V. Florey, 'Vitamin–mineral supplementation and intelligence', *Lancet*, 336, 1990, 175.

10 S. J. Schoenthaler, S. P. Amos, H. J. Eysenck, E. Peritz and J. Yudkin, 'Controlled trial of vitamin–mineral supplementation effects on intelligence and performance', *Personality and Individual Differences*, 12, 1991, 351–62.

11 ibid., p. 351.

12 ibid.; S. Schoenthaler, personal communication, 1995.

13 *Daily Telegraph*, 22 Feb. 1988.

14 J. Yudkin, 'Intelligence of children and vitamin–mineral supplements: the DRF study. Discussion, conclusion and consequences', *Personality and Individual Differences*, 12, 1991, 363–5.

15 R. G. Whitehead, 'Vitamins, minerals, schoolchildren and IQ', *British Medical Journal*, 302, 1991, 548.

16 *The Diets of British Schoolchildren*, Department of Health Report 36, London, HMSO, 1989.

17 R. Griffiths and D. Benton, 'The impact of vitamin–mineral supplementation on the attention and intelligence scores of an eight-year-old boy – a case study', *Journal of Nutritional Medicine*, 4, 1994, 87–94.

18 Anonymous, 'Brains and vitamins', *Lancet*, 337, 1991, 587–8; Whitehead, *British Medical Journal*, 302, 1991, 548.

19 Whitehead, *British Medical Journal*, 302, 1991, 548.

20 P. Aldhous, 'IQ data controversy', *Nature*, 350, 1991, 5.

21 Benton and Cook, *Lancet*, i, 1988, 140–43; Schoenthaler *et al.*, *Personality and Individual Differences*, 12, 1991, 343–50; Nelson *et al.*, *British Journal of Nutrition*, 64, 1990, 13–22; Crombie *et al.*, *Lancet*, 335, 1990, 744–7; Benton and Buts, *Lancet*, 335, 1990, 1158–60; Schoenthaler *et al.*, *Personality and Individual Differences*, 12, 1991, 351–62; S. Southon, A. J. A. Wright, P. M. Finglas *et al.*, 'Dietary intake and micronutrient status of adolescents: effect of vitamin and trace element supplementation on indices of status and performance in tests of verbal and non-verbal intelligence', *British Journal of Nutrition*, 71, 1994, 897–918; M. G.

Kerimova and I. G. Aleskerova, 'Influence of ration correction and varying doses of glutamevitum on the vitamin status and working capacity of children attending school from the age of six' (in Russian), *Voprosy Pitaniia*, 1990, 30–34; S. I. Nidich, P. Morehead, R. J. Nidich, D. Sands and H. Sharma, 'The effect of the Maharishi Rasayana food supplement on non-verbal intelligence', *Personality and Individual Differences*, 15, 1993, 599–602; D. Benton and R. Cook, 'Vitamin and mineral supplements improve the intelligence scores and concentration of six-year-old children', *Personality and Individual Differences*, 12, 1991, 1151–8.

## 5. Food Allergy or Food Intolerance?

1 R. Mackarness, *Not All in the Mind*, London, Pan, 1976.

2 A. H. Rowe, *Food Allergy, Its Manifestations, Diagnosis and Treatment with a General Discussion of Bronchial Asthma*, Philadelphia, Lee and Febiger, 1931.

3 A. F. Coca, *Familial Nonreaginic Food-Allergy*, Springfield, Ill., Charles C. Thomas, 1942.

4 T. G. Randolph, H. J. Rinkel and M. Zeller, *Food Allergy*, Springfield, Ill., Charles C. Thomas, 1951.

5 Mackarness, *Not All in the Mind*, p. 24.

6 D. J. Pearson, 'Problems with terminology and with study design in food sensitivity', in J. Dobbing (ed.), *Food Intolerance*, London, Bailliere Tindall, 1987.

7 D. J. Pearson, K. J. B. Rix and S. J. Bentley, 'Food Allergy. How much in the mind?', *Lancet*, 1, 1983, 1259–61.

8 Ministry of Agriculture, Fisheries and Food, *Mites in Stored Commodities*, MAFF Advisory Leaflet 489, London, HMSO, 1974.

9 H. M. G. Doeglas, J. Huisman and J. P. Nater, 'Histamine intoxication after cheese', *Lancet*, 2, 1967, 1361–2.

10 S. L. Rice, R. Eitenmiller and P. E. Koehler, 'Biologically active amines in food: a review', *Journal of Milk and Food Technology*, 39, 1976, 353–8.

11 J. D. Johnson, 'The regional and ethnic distribution of lactose malabsorption. Adaptive and genetic hypothesis', in I. M. Paige and T. M. Bayless (eds.), *Lactose Digestion*, Baltimore, Md, Johns Hopkins University Press, 1981.

12 A. Ferguson, D. M. MacDonald and W. G. Brydon, 'Prevalence of lactase deficiency in British adults', *Gut*, 25, 1984, 163–7.

13 M. H. Lessof, D. G. Wraith, T. G. Merrett, J. Merrett and P. D.

Buisseret, 'Food allergy and intolerance in 100 patients in local and systemic effects', *Quarterly Journal of Medicine*, 49, 1980, 259–71.

14 'Food Intolerance and Food Aversion. A joint report of the Royal College of Physicians and the British Nutrition Foundation', *Journal of the Royal College of Physicians*, 18, 1984, 3–41.

15 ibid.

16 Mackarness, *Not All in the Mind*.

17 D. J. Pearson, K. J. B. Rix and S. J. Bentley, 'Food allergy: How much in the mind?', *Lancet*, i, 1983, 1259–61.

## 6. Hyperactivity: A Reaction to Additives?

1 H. Hoffman, *Der Struwelpeter oder lustige Geschichten und drollige Bilder*, Leipzig, Insel Verlag, 1844. Quoted by J. Egger, 'The Hyperkinetic Syndrome', in J. Brostoff and S. J. Challacombe (eds.), *Food Allergy and Intolerance*, London, Bailliere Tindall, 1987.

2 Mintel, *Additives and the Consumer*, London, Mintel, 1987.

3 F. Lawrence (ed.), *Additives – Your Complete Survival Guide*, London, Century, 1986.

4 B. F. Feingold, *Why Your Child Is Hyperactive*, New York, Random House, 1975.

5 ibid.

6 B. F. Feingold, 'Hyperkinesis and learning disabilities linked to artificial food flavours and colors', *American Journal of Nursing*, 75, 1975, 797–803.

7 C. K. Conners, C. H. Goyette, D. A. Southwick, J. M. Lees, and P. A. Andrulonis, 'Food additives and hyperkinesis: a controlled double-blind experiment', *Pediatrics*, 2, 1976, 154–66.

8 V. Rippere, 'Food additives and hyperactive children: a critique of Conners', *British Journal of Clinical Psychology*, 22, 1983, 19–32.

9 J. M. Swanson and M. Kinsbourne, 'Food dyes impair performance of hyperactive children on a laboratory learning test', *Science*, 207, 1980, 1485–7.

10 National Advisory Committee on Hyperkinesis and Food Additives, *Final Report to the Nutrition Foundation*, New York, The Nutrition Foundation, 1980.

11 K. A. Kavale and S. R. Forness, 'Hyperactivity and diet treatment: a meta-analysis of the Feingold hypothesis', *Journal of Learning Disabilities*, 16, 1983, 324–30.

12 J. A. Mattes, 'The Feingold diet: a current reappraisal', *Journal of Learning Disabilities*, 16, 1983, 319-23.

13 J. Egger, 'The hyperkinetic syndrome', in J. Brostoff and S. J. Challacombe (eds.), *Food Allergy and Intolerance*, London, Bailliere Tindall, 1987.

14 B. Rimland, 'The Feingold diet: an assessment of the reviews by Mattes, by Kavale and Forness and others', *Journal of Learning Disabilities* 16, 1983, 331-3.

15 J. Egger, C. M. Carter, J. Wilson, M. W. Turner and J. F. Soothill, 'Is migraine food allergy? A double-blind controlled trial of oligoantigenic diet treatment', *Lancet*, ii, 1983, 865-9.

16 ibid.

17 J. Egger, C. M. Carter, P. J. Graham, D. Gumley and J. F. Soothill, 'Controlled trial of oligoantigenic treatment in the hyperkinetic syndrome', *Lancet*, 14, 1985, 540-45.

18 P. Marshall, 'Attention deficit disorder and allergy: a neurochemical model of the relation between the illnesses', *Psychological Bulletin*, 106, 1989, 434-46.

19 C. M. Carter, M. Urabowicz, R. Hemsley, *et al.*, 'Effect of a new food diet in attention deficit disorder', *Archives of Disease in Childhood*, 69, 1993, 564-8.

## 7. Glucose: the Food of the Brain

1 W. Duffy, *Sugar Blues*, Radnor, Pa, Chilton, 1975.

2 S. R. Buchanan, 'The most ubiquitous toxin', *American Psychologist*, 39, 1984, 1327-8.

3 J. Yudkin, *Pure White and Deadly*, Harmondsworth, Penguin, 1972.

4 I. J. Deary, S. J. Langan, K. S. Graham, D. Hepburn and B. M. Frier, 'Recurrent severe hypoglycemia intelligence and speed of information processing', *Intelligence*, 16, 1992, 337-57.

5 S. Harris, 'Hyperinsulinism and dysinsulinism', *Journal of the American Medical Association*, 83, 1924, 729.

6 Duffy, *Sugar Blues*.

7 V. Marks and F. G. Rose, *Hypoglycaemia* (2nd edn), Oxford, Blackwell Scientific Publications, 1981.

8 A. Lev-Ran and R. W. Anderson, 'The diagnosis of postprandial hypoglycemia', *Diabetes*, 30, 1981, 996-9.

9 K. G. M. Alberti, A. Dornhorst and A. S. Rowe, 'Metabolic rhythms in

normal and diabetic man', *Israel Journal of Medical Science*, 11, 1975, 571–80.

10 D. Benton and D. Owens, 'Is raised blood glucose associated with the relief of tension?', *Journal of Psychosomatic Research*, 37, 1993, 723–35.

11 D. S. Owens, P. Y. Parker and D. Benton, Blood glucose influences mood following demanding cognitive tasks, Submitted for publication.

12 J. D. Brooke, S. Toogood and L. F. Green, 'Diet, physiological work and accident incidence of forge workers', *Scandinavian Journal of Work and Environmental Health*, 6, 1980, 66–72.

13 J. Keul, G. Huber, M. Lehmann, A. Berg and E. F. Jakob, 'Einfluß von Dextrose auf Fahrleistung, Konzentrationsfahigkeit, Kreislauf und Stoffwechsel im Kraftfahrzeug-Simulator (Doppelblindstudie im cross-over-design)', *Aktuelle Ernährungsmedizin*, Georg Thieme Verlag 7, 1982, 7–14.

14 M. S. Christian, Letter, *British Medical Journal*, ii, 1972, 295.

15 Keul *et al.*, *Aktuelle Ernährungsmedizin*, 7, 1982, 7–14.

16 O. Snorgaard, L. H. Lassen, A. M. Rosenfalck and C. Binder, 'Glycaemic thresholds for hypoglycaemic symptoms impairment of cognitive function and release of counter regulatory hormones in subjects with functional hypoglycaemia', *Journal of Internal Medicine*, 229, 1991, 343–50.

17 Personal correspondence, 24 Feb. 1991.

18 W. G. Crook, 'An alternative method of managing the hyperactive child', *Pediatrics*, 54, 1974, 656.

19 R. J. Prinz, W. A. Roberts and E. Hantman, 'Dietary correlates of hyperactive behavior in children', *Journal of Consulting and Clinical Psychology*, 48, 1980, 760–69.

20 R. J. Prinz and D. B. Riddle, 'Association between nutrition and behavior in five-year-old children', *Nutrition Reviews*, 44 Supplement, 1986, 151–8.

21 Prinz *et al.*, *Journal of Consulting and Clinical Psychology*, 48, 1980, 760–69.

22 D. Connors, K. Wells, W. Horn, *et al.*, 'The effects of sucrose and fructose on behavior of child psychiatric patients', Sugar Associates Inc. report, 1982.

23 D. Behar, J. L. Rapoport, A. J. Adams, C. J. Berg and M. Cornblath, 'Sugar challenge testing with children considered behaviorally "sugar reactive"', *Nutrition and Behavior*, 1, 1984 277–88.

24 L. K. Mahan, M. Chase, C. T. Furukawa, *et al.*, 'Sugar "allergy" and children's behavior', paper given at the 41st Annual Meeting of the American Academy of Allergy and Immunology, New York, 1985.

25 ibid.

26 M. D. Gross, 'Effect of sucrose on hyperkinetic children', *Pediatrics*, 74, 1984, 876–8.

27 D. J. Rapp, 'Does diet affect hyperactivity?', *Learning Disabilities*, 11, 1978, 383–9.

28 M. J. P. Kreusi, J. L. Rapoport, M. Cummings, *et al.*, 'Effects of sugar and aspartame on aggression and activity in children', *American Journal of Psychiatry*, 144, 1987, 1487–90.

29 R. Walton, R. Hudak and R. J. Green-Waite, 'Adverse reactions to aspartame: double-blind challenge in patients from a vulnerable population', *Biological Psychiatry*, 34, 1993, 13–17.

30 J. Egger, C. M. Carter, P. J. Graham, D. Gumley and J. F. Soothill, 'Controlled trial of oligoantigenic treatment in the hyperkinetic syndrome', *Lancet*, 14, 1985, 540–45.

31 P. A. Crapo, G. Reaven and J. Olefsky, 'Postprandial plasma-glucose and insulin response to different complex carbohydrates', *Diabetes*, 26, 1977, 1178–83.

32 Department of Health, *Dietary sugars and human disease*, Department of Health Report on Health and Social Subjects, vol. 37, London, HMSO, 1989.

33 D. Benton and R. Cook, 'Vitamin and mineral suplements improve the intelligence scores and concentration of six-year-old children', *Personality and Individual Differences*, 12, 1991, 1151–8.

34 ibid.

35 Department of Health, *Dietary sugars*.

## 8. Diet and Violence

1 *Guardian*, 5 Sept. 1988.

2 US Select Committee on Nutrition and Human Needs, *Diet related to killer diseases, V: nutrition and mental health*, Washington, DC, US Government Printing Office, 1977.

3 A. Schauss, *Diet crime and delinquency*, New York, Random House, 1980.

4 W. G. Crook, 'Can what a child eats make him dull, stupid or hyperactive?', *Journal of Learning Disabilities*, 13, 1980, 53–8.

5 Personal correspondence.

6 Personal correspondence.

7 P. Pelto, 'Psychological anthropology', in A. Beals and B. Stegel (eds.),

*Biennial Review of Anthropology*, Stanford, Calif., Stanford University Press, 1967, p. 151.

8 R. Bolton, 'Aggression and hypoglycaemia among the Qolla: a study in psycho-biological anthropology', *Ethnology*, 12, 1973, 227–57.

9 R. Bolton, 'Hostility in fantasy: a further test of the hypoglycaemia–aggression hypothesis', *Aggressive Behavior*, 2, 1976, 257–74.

10 ibid.; Bolton, *Ethnology*, 12, 1973, 227–57.

11 M. Virkkunen, and M. O. Huttunen, 'Evidence for abnormal glucose tolerance among violent offenders', *Neuropsychobiology*, 8, 1982, 30–34.

12 M. Virkkunnen, 'Insulin secretion during the glucose tolerance test among habitually violent and impulsive offenders', *Aggressive Behavior*, 12, 1986, 303–10.

13 ibid.

14 D. Benton, N. Kumari and P. F. Brain, 'Mild hypoglycemia and questionnaire measures of aggression,' *Biological Psychology*, 14, 1982, 129–35.

15 D. Benton, V. Brett, P. F. Brain, 'Glucose improves attention and the reaction to frustration in children', *Biological Psychology*, 24, 1987, 95–100.

16 D. Benton and D. Owens, 'Is high blood glucose associated with feeling relaxed?', *Journal of Psychosomatic Research*, 37, 1993, 723–35.

17 S. Schoenthaler, 'Diet and crime: An empirical examination of the value of nutrition in the control and treatment of incarcerated juvenile offenders', *International Journal of Biosocial Research*, 4, 1983, 25–39.

18 S. Schoenthaler, 'Malnutrition and maladaptive behavior: two correlational analyses and a double-blind placebo-controlled challenge in five states', in W. B. Essman, (ed.), *Nutrients and Brain Function*, Basel, Karger, 1987, pp. 198–218.

19 S. J. Schoenthaler, 'The northern California diet-behavior program: an empirical examination of 3000 incarcerated juveniles in Stanislaus County juvenile hall', *International Journal of Biosocial Research*, 5, 1983, 99–106.

20 S. J. Schoenthaler, 'Controlled trial of vitamin–mineral supplementation on institutional violence and anti-social behavior', *Personality and Individual Differences*, 12, 1991, 340.

21 S. J. Schoenthaler and S. Amos, A controlled trial of vitamin–mineral supplementation within the California Youth Authority: The effect on institutional violence and antisocial behavior. (Personal communication.)

22 *Independent*, 27 Nov. 1989.

23 'Statement of the Ad Hoc Committee on Hypoglycaemia', *Annual of Internal Medicine*, 78, 1973, 300–301.

## 9. Too Little or Too Much of a Good Thing?

1 L. Pauling, 'Orthomolecular psychiatry', *Science*, 160, 1968, 265–71.

2 R. J. Williams, *Biochemical Individuality*, New York, John Wiley, 1956.

3 J. Brozek, 'Psychological effects of thiamine restriction and deprivation in normal young men', *American Journal of Clinical Nutrition*, 5, 1957, 109–18.

4 W. W. Tuttle, M. Wilson, K. Deaaum and H. Rhodes, 'Influence of various levels of thiamine intake on physiologic response', *Journal of the American Dietetics Association*, 25, 1949, 21–7.

5 H. E. de Wardener and B. Lennox, 'Cerebral Beriberi (Wernicke's Encephalopathy)', *Lancet*, i, 1947, 11–17.

6 R. F. Harrell, 'Mental response to added thiamine', *Journal of Nutrition*, 31, 1946 283–98.

7 L. J. Smidt, F. M. Cremin, L. E. Grivetti and A. J. Clifford, 'Influence of thiamin supplementation on the health and general well-being of an elderly Irish population with marginal thiamin deficiency', *Journal of Gerontology*, 46, 1991, M16–M22.

8 A. Nadel and P. C. Burger, 'Wernicke Encephalopathy following prolonged intravenous therapy', *Journal of the American Medical Association*, 235, 1976, 2403–5.

9 Editorial, 'Korsakoff's syndrome', *Lancet*, 336, 1990, 912–13.

10 C. Harper, 'The incidence of Wernicke's encephalopathy in Australia – a neuropathological study of 131 cases', *Journal of Neurology, Neurosurgery and Psychiatry*, 46, 1983, 593–8.

11 J. Price, R. Kerr, M. Hicks and P. F. Nixon, 'The Wernicke-Korsakoff syndrome: a reappraisal in Queensland with special reference to prevention', *Medical Journal of Australia*, 147, 1987, 561–5.

12 D. Lonsdale and R. J. Shamburger, 'Red cell transketolase as an indicator of nutritional deficiency', *American Journal of Clinical Nutrition*, 33, 1980, 205–11.

13 M. W. P. Carney, A. Ravindran, M. Rinsler and D. G. Williams, 'Thiamine, riboflavin and pyridoxine deficiency in psychiatric patients', *British Journal of Psychiatry*, 135, 1982, 249–54.

14 R. T. Sterner and R. W. Price, 'Restricted riboflavin: within subject behavioral effects in humans', *American Journal of Clinical Nutrition*, 26, 1973, 150–60.

15 M. W. P. Carney, 'Vitamin deficiency and mental symptoms', *British Journal of Psychiatry*, 156, 1990, 878–82.

16 S. M. Loriaux, J. B. Deijen, J. F. Orlebeke and J. H. De Swart, 'The

effects of nicotinic acid and xanthinol nicotinate on human memory in different categories of age', *Psychopharmacology*, 87, 1985, 390–95.

17 A. Hoffer and H. Osmond, 'Nicotinamide Adenine Dinucleotide (NAD) as a treatment for schizophrenia', *Journal of Psychopharmacology*, 1, 1966, 79–95.

18 L. R. Mosher, 'Nicotinic acid side effects and toxicity: a review', *American Journal of Psychiatry*, 126, 1979, 124–30.

19 American Psychiatric Association, 'Megavitamin and orthomolecular therapy in psychiatry', *Nutrition Reviews*, 32, Supplement, 1974, 44–7.

20 H. Sauberlich and J. Canham, 'Vitamin $B_6$', in R. Goodhart and M. Shils, *Modern Nutrition in Health and Disease*, Philadelphia, Lea and Febiger, 1980.

21 J. Kleijnen and P. Knipschild, 'Niacin and vitamin $B_6$ in mental functioning: a review of controlled trials in humans', *Biological Psychiatry*, 29, 1991, 931–41.

22 J. B. Deijen, E. J. van der Beek, J. F. Orlebeke and H. van den Berg, 'Vitamin $B_6$ supplementation in elderly men: effects on mood, memory performance and mental effort', *Psychopharmacology*, 109, 1992, 489–96.

23 A. G. Heeley and G. E. Roberts, 'A study of tryptophan metabolism in psychotic children', *Developmental Medicine and Child Neurology*, 3, 1966, 708–18.

24 J. Noakes, letter to the *Observer*, 1966.

25 B. Rimland, E. Callaway and P. Dreyfus, 'The effect of high doses of vitamin $B_6$ on autistic children: a double-blind crossover study', *American Journal of Psychiatry*, 135, 1978, 472–5.

26 C. Barthelemy, B. Garreau, I. Leddet, *et al.*, 'Behavioral and biological effects of oral magnesium, vitamin $B_6$ and combined magnesium–vitamin $B_6$ administration in autistic children', *Magnesium Bulletin*, 2, 1981, 150–53; J. Martineau, C. Barthelemy, B. Garreau and G. LeLord, 'Vitamin $B_6$ magnesium and combined $B_6$-Mg: Therapeutic effects in childhood autism', *Biological Psychiatry*, 20, 1985, 462–75.

27 B. Rimland, 'The use of megavitamin $B_6$ and magnesium in the treatment of autistic children and adults', *Institute for Child Behavior Research*, Publication Number 73, 1986.

28 II. Schaumburg, J. Kaplan, A Windebank, *et al.*, 'Sensory neuropathy from pyridoxine abuse: a new megavitamin syndrome', *New England Journal of Medicine*, 309, 1983, 445–8.

29 C. J. Farmer, 'Some aspects of vitamin C metabolism', *Federation Proceedings*, 3, 1944, 179.

30 R. H. Kinsman and J. Hood, 'Some behavioral effects of ascorbic acid deficiency', *American Journal of Clinical Nutrition*, 24, 1971, 455–64.

31 A. L. Kubula and M. M. Katz, 'Nutritional factors in psychological test behavior', *Journal of Genetic Psychology*, 96, 1960, 343–52.

32 S. Southon, A. J. A. Wright, P. M. Finglas *et al.*, 'Dietary intake and micronutrient status of adolescents: effect of vitamin and trace element supplementation on indices of status and performance in tests of verbal and non-verbal intelligence', *British Journal of Nutrition*, 71, 1994, 897–918.

33 S. O. Kayaalp, J. S. Rubenstein and N. H. Neff, 'Inhibition of dopamine D-1 and D-2 binding sites in neuronal tissue by ascorbate', *Neuropharmacology*, 20, 1981, 409–10.

34 D. Benton, 'The influence of large doses of Vitamin C on psychological functioning', *Psychopharmacology*, 75, 1981, 98–9.

35 G. J. Naylor and A. H. W. Smith, 'Vanadium: a possible aetiological factor in manic depressive illness', *Psychological Medicine*, 11, 1981, 249–56.

36 A. Cott, 'Megavitamins. The orthomolecular approach to behaviour disorders and learning disabilities', *Academic Therapy*, VII, 1972, 245–58.

37 R. F. Harrell, R. H. Capp, D. R. Davis, *et al.*, 'Can nutritional supplements help mentally retarded children? An exploratory study', *Proceedings of the National Academy of Sciences*, 78, 1981, 574–8.

38 ibid.

39 B.W. Kozlowski, 'Megavitamin treatment of mental retardation in children: a review of effects of behavior and cognition', *Journal of Child and Adolescent Psychopharmacology*, 2, 1992, 307–20.

40 ibid.

41 A. Brenner, 'The effects of megadoses of selected B complex vitamins on children with hyperkinesis: controlled studies with long-term follow up', *Journal of Learning Disabilities*, 15, 1982, 258–64.

42 J. Marks, 'The safety of the vitamins: an overview', in P. Walter, H. Stahelin and G. Brubacher, (eds.), *Elevated Dosages of Vitamins*, Toronto, Hans Huber, 1989, 12–24.

43 Schaumburg *et al.*, *New England Journal of Medicine*, 309, 1983, 445–8.

44 K.-H. Bassler, 'Use and abuse of high dosages of vitamin $B_6$', in P. Walter, H. Stahelin and G. Brubacher (eds.), *Elevated Dosages of Vitamins*, Toronto, Hans Huber, 1989, 120–26.

45 J. M. Rivers, 'Safety of high-level vitamin C ingestion', in P. Walter, H. Stahelin and G. Brubacher (eds.), *Elevated Dosages of Vitamins*, Toronto, Hans Huber, 1989, 95–108.

## 10. Can Diet Slow Ageing?

1 Department of Health and Social Security, *A Nutrition Survey of the Elderly*, Report of Health Social Subjects No. 3, London, HMSO, 1972.

2 B. S. Worthington-Roberts and W. R. Hazzard, 'Nutrition and Aging', *Annual Review of Gerontology and Geriatrics*, 3, 1982, 297–328.

3 J. S. Goodwin, J. M. Goodwin and P. J. Garry, 'Association between nutritional status and cognitive functioning in a healthy elderly population', *Journal of the American Medical Association*, 249, 1983, 2917–21.

4 G. F. Taylor, 'A clinical survey of elderly people from a nutritional standpoint', in A. N. Exton-Smith and D. L. Scott (eds.), *Vitamins in the Elderly*, Bristol, John Wright, 1968.

5 L. J. Smidt, F. M. Cremin, L. E. Grivetti and A. J. Clifford, 'Influence of thiamin supplementation on the health and general well-being of an elderly Irish population with marginal thiamin deficiency', *Journal of Gerontology*, 46, 1991, M16–M22.

6 For example, M. W. P. Carney and M. T. Sheffield, 'Serum folic acid and $B_{12}$ in 272 psychiatric inpatients', *Psychological Medicine*, 8, 1978, 139–44.

7 M. Hector and J. R. Burton, 'What are the psychiatric manifestations of vitamin $B_{12}$ deficiency?', *Journal of the American Geriatric Society*, 36, 1988, 1105–12.

8 I. R. Bell, J. S. Edman, D. W. Marby, A. Satlin, T. Dreier, B. Liptzin and J. O. Cole, 'Vitamin $B_{12}$ and folate status in acute geropsychiatric inpatients: affective and cognitive characteristics of a vitamin nondeficient population', *Biological Psychiatry*, 27, 1990, 125–37.

9 Carney and Sheffield, *Psychological Medicine*, 8, 1978, 139–44.

10 R. Doll, 'Review: Alzheimer's disease and environmental aluminium', *Age and Ageing*, 22, 1993, 138–53.

11 D. R. McLachlan, P. E. Fraser and A. J. Dalton, 'Aluminium and the pathogenesis of Alzheimer's disease: a summary of evidence', *IBA Foundation Symposium*, 169, 1992, 87–108.

12 R. T. Bartus, R. L. Dean, B. Beer and A. S. Lippa, 'The cholinergic hypothesis of geriatric memory dysfunction', *Science*, 217, 1982, 408–17.

13 K. M. Perryman and L. J. Fitten, 'Delayed matching to sample performance during a double-blind trial of tacrine and lecithin in patients with Alzheimer's disease', *Life Science*, 53, 1993, 479–86.

14 M. Dysken, 'A review of recent clinical trials in the treatment of Alzheimer's Dementia', *Psychiatric Annals*, 17, 1987, 178–91.

15 C. Messier, T. Durkin, O. Mrabet and C. Destrade, 'Memory-improving action of glucose: indirect evidence for a facilitation of hippocampal

acetylcholine synthesis', *Behavioural Brain Research*, 39, 1990, 135–43; T. P. Durkin, C. Messier, P. de Boer and B. H. C. Westerink, 'Raised glucose levels enhance scopolamine-induced acetylcholine overflow from the hippocampus: an *in vivo* microdialysis study in the rat', *Behavioural Brain Research*, 49, 1992, 181–8.

16 For example, C. A. Manning, J. L. Hall and P. E. Gold, 'Glucose effects on memory and other neuropsychological tests in elderly humans', *Psychological Science*, 1, 1990, 307–11.

17 ibid.; S. Craft, G. Zallen and L. D. Baker, 'Glucose and memory in mild senile dementia of the Alzheimer type', *Journal of Clinical and Experimental Neuropsychology*, 14, 1992, 253–67.

18 P. R. Borum, 'Carnitine', *Annual Review of Nutrition*, 3, 1983, 233–59.

19 C. A. Barnes, A. L. Markowska, D. K. Ingram, *et al.*, 'Acetyl-l-carnitine: effects on learning and memory performance of aged rats in simple and complex mazes', *Neurobiology of Aging*, 11, 1990, 499–506.

20 R. Lucreziotti, O. Ghirardi, M. T. Ramacci and F. Amenti, 'Improved morphology of aged rat brain by L-acetylcarnitine', *Neuroscience Letters*, 14, 1983, S225.

21 A. L. Markowska, D. K. Ingram, C. A. Barnes *et al.*, 'Acetyl-l-carnitine 1: effects on mortality pathology and sensory-motor performance in aging rats', *Neurobiology of Aging*, 11, 1990, 491–8.

22 D. Cucinotta, M. Passeri, S. Ventura, *et al.*, 'Multicenter clinical placebo-controlled study with acetyl-l-carnitine in the treatment of mildly demented elderly patients', *Drug Development Research*, 14, 1988, 213–16.

23 R. Weindruch, P. H. Naylor, A. L. Goldstein and R. L. Walford, 'The retardation of aging in mice by dietary restriction: longevity, cancer, immunity and lifetime energy intake', *Journal of Nutrition*, 116, 1989, 641.

24 S. N. Austrad, 'Life extension by dietary restriction in the bowl and doily spider, *Frontinella pyramitela*', *Experimental Gerontology*, 24, 1989, 83–92.

25 E. A. Vallejo, 'La dieta de hambre a dias alternos in la alimentacion de los viejos', *Revista Clinica Espanola*, 63, 1957, 25.

26 E. J. M. Velthuis-te Wierik and H. van den Berg, 'Energy restriction the basis for successful aging in man?', *Nutrition Research*, 14, 1994, 1113–34.

27 ibid.

28 R. Weindruch and R. L. Walford, *The Retardation of Aging and Disease by Dietary Restriction*, Springfield, Ill., C. C. Thomas, 1988.

29 D. Harman, 'Free radical involvement in aging', *Drugs and Aging*, 3, 1993, 60–80.

## 11. Diet and Mood

1 J. D. Fernstrom and R. J. Wurtman, 'Brain serotonin content: physiological regulation by plasma neutral amino acids', *Science*, 178, 1972, 414–16.

2 P. Willner, *Depression: A Psychobiological Synthesis*, New York, John Wiley, 1985.

3 R. J. Wurtman and J. J. Wurtman, 'Carbohydrates and depression', *Scientific American*, Jan. 1989, 68–75.

4 Quoted ibid.

5 ibid.

6 Fernstrom and Wurtman, *Science*, 178, 1972, 414–16.

7 N. Rosenthal, M. Genhart, B. Caballero, *et al.*, 'Psychological effects of carbohydrate- and protein-rich meals in patients with seasonal affective disorder', *Biological Psychiatry*, 25, 1989, 1029–40.

8 J. J. Wurtman, A. Brzezinski, R. J. Wurtman and B. Laferrere, 'Effect of nutrient intake on premenstrual depression', *American Journal of Obstetrics and Gynecology*, 161, 1989, 1228–34.

9 ibid.

10 D. J. Bowen and N. E. Grunberg, 'Variation in food preference and consumption across the menstrual cycle', *Physiology and Behavior*, 47, 1990, 287–91.

11 S. P. Dalvit-McPhillips, 'The effect of the human menstrual cycle on nutrient intake', *Physiology and Behavior*, 31, 1983, 209–12.

12 B. J. Spring, H. R. Lieberman, G. Swope and G. S. Garfield, 'Effects of carbohydrates on mood and behavior', *Nutrition Reviews*, 44 (Suppl), 1986, 51–60.

13 J. D. Fernstrom, 'Tryptophan serotonin and carbohydrate appetite: will the real carbohydrate craver please stand up?', *Journal of Nutrition*, 118, 1988, 1417–19.

14 M. F. Muldoon, S. B. Manuck and K. A. Matthews, 'Lowering cholesterol concentrations and mortality: a quantitative review of primary prevention trials', *British Medical Journal*, 310, 1990, 309–14.

15 J. R. Kaplan, S. B. Manuck and C. Shively, 'The effect of fat and cholesterol on social behavior in monkeys', *Psychosomatic Medicine*, 53, 1991, 634–42.

16 M. Virkunnen and H. Pentinnen, 'Serum cholesterol in aggressive conduct disorder: a preliminary study', *Biological Psychiatry*, 19, 1984, 435–9.

17 G. Lindberg, L. Rastam, B. Gullberg and G. A. Ekland, 'Low serum

cholesterol concentration and short term mortality from injuries in men and women', *British Medical Journal*, 305, 1992, 277–9.

18 C. J. Glueck, M. Tieger, R. Kunkel, *et al.*, 'Hypocholesterolemia and affective disorder', *American Journal of Medical Sciences*, 308, 1994, 218–25.

19 H. Engelberg, 'Low serum cholesterol and suicide', *Lancet*, 339, 1992, 727–9.

20 D. Benton, 'Do low cholesterol levels slow mental processing?', *Psychosomatic Medicine*, 57, 1995, 50–53.

21 J. C. Millichap, J. C. Jones and B. P. Rudis, 'Mechanisms of anticonvulsant action of ketogenic diet', *American Journal of Disorders of Children*, 107, 1964, 593–604.

22 Benton, *Psychosomatic Medicine*, 57, 1995, 50–53.

23 D. Benton, J. Haller and J. Fordy, 'Vitamin supplementation for one year improves mood', *Neuropsychobiology*, 32, 1995, 98–105.

24 H. Heseker, W. Kubler, J. Westenhoefer and V. Pudel, 'Psychische Veranderungen als Fruhzeichen einer suboptimalen Vitaminversorgung', *Ernahrungsumschau*, 37, 1990, 87–94.

25 A. Bendich and C. E. Butterworth, *Micronutrients in Health and in Disease Prevention*, New York, Marcel Dekker, 1991.

26 Benton *et al.*, *Neuropsycholobiology*, 32, 1995, 98–105.

27 D. A. Bender, *Nutritional Biochemistry of the Vitamins*, Cambridge, Cambridge University Press, 1992.

28 J. Kleijnen, G. ter Riet and P. Knipschild, 'Vitamin $B_6$ in the treatment of the premenstrual syndrome – a review', *British Journal of Obstetrics and Gynaecology*, 97, 1990, 847–52.

29 P. W. Adams, D. P. Rose, J. Folkard, *et al.*, 'Effect of pyridoxine hydrochloride upon depression associated with oral contraceptives', *Lancet*, i, 1973, 897–904.

30 S. Yehuda and M. B. H. Youdim, 'Brain iron deficiency: biochemistry and behaviour', in M. B. H. Youdim (ed.), *Brain Iron: Neurochemical and Behavioural Aspects*, London, Taylor and Francis, 1988, pp. 89–114.

31 J. Fordy and D. Benton, 'Does low iron status influence psychological functioning?', *Journal of Human Nutrition and Dietetics*, 7, 1994, 127–33.

32 ibid.

33 D. Benton and R. Cook, 'The impact of selenium supplementation on mood', *Biological Psychiatry*, 29, 1991, 1092–8.

34 J. Thorn, J. Robertson and D. H. Buss, 'Trace nutrients: selenium in British food', *British Journal of Nutrition*, 39, 1978, 391–6.

35 M. I. Barclay and A. MacPherson, 'Selenium content of wheat flour used in the UK', *Journal of the Science of Food and Agriculture*, 37, 1986, 1133–8.

36 J. R. Arthur, F. Nicol and J. Beckett, 'Hepatic iodothyronine 5-deiodinase', *Biochemical Journal*, 272, 1990, 537–40.

## 12. Meals and the Way You Think

1 A. P. Smith and A. Kendrick, 'Meals and performance', in A. P. Smith and D. M. Jones (eds.), *Handbook of Human Performance*, vol. 2, London, Academic Press, 1992, pp. 1–23.

2 D. Benton and P. Y. Parker, Breakfast, blood glucose and cognition', *Journal of the American Dietetics Association*, in press.

3 S. Folkard and T. H. Monk (eds.), *Hours of Work: Temporal Factors in Work Scheduling*, Chicester, Wiley, 1985.

4 Smith and Kendrick, *Handbook of Human Performance*.

5 ibid.

6 A. P. Smith, S. Leekham, A. Ralph and G. McNeill, 'The influence of meal composition on post-lunch changes in performance efficiency and mood', *Appetite*, 10, 1988, 195–203.

7 H. M. Lloyd, M. W. Green and P. J. Rogers, 'Mood and cognitive performance effects of isocaloriac lunches differing in fat and carbohydrate content', *Physiology and Behavior*, 56, 1994, 51–7.

8 A. Keys, J. Brozek, A. Henschel, O. Mickelson and H. L. Taylor, *The Biology. of Human Starvation*, vol. 2, Minneapolis, University of Minnesota Press, 1950.

9 M. W. Green, P. J. Rogers, N. A. Elliman and S. J. Gatenby, 'Impairment of cognitive performance associated with dieting and high levels of dietary restraint', *Physiology and Behaviour*, 55, 1994, 447–52.

10 M. W. Green, N. A. Elliman and P. J. Rogers, 'Lack of effect of short-term fasting on cognitive function', *Journal of Psychiatric Research*, 29, 1995, 245–53.

11 R. G. Laessle, S. Bossert, G. Hank, K. Halweg and K. M. Pirke, 'Cognitive performance in patients with bulimia nervosa: relationship to intermittent starvation', *Biological Psychiatry*, 27, 1990, 549–51.

12 D. Benton, 'Lipids and cognitive functioning', in M. Hillbrand and R.T. Spitz, (eds.), *Lipids and Human Behavior*, Washington, DC, American Psychological Association, 1996.

13 J. C. Millichap, J. C. Jones and B. P. Rudis, 'Mechanisms of anticonvulsant action of ketogenic diet', *American Journal of Disorders of Childhood*, 107, 1964, 593–604.

14 R. Cook and D. Benton, 'The relationship between diet and mental health', *Personality and Individual Differences*, 14, 1993, 397–403.

15 H. P. Weingarten and D. Elston, 'Food cravings in a college population', *Appetite*, 17, 1991, 167–75.

16 M. Roach, 'More reasons to love chocolate', *New Woman*, Feb. 1989, 135–6.

17 Cadbury Ltd, 'Sales of chocolate confectionery in the UK, 1981–1991', *Chocolate Market Review*, Bournville, England, Cadbury Ltd, 1991.

18 C. A. Shively and S. M. Tarka, 'Methylxanthine composition and consumption patterns of cocoa and chocolate products', in G.A. Spiller (ed.), *The Methylxanthine Beverages and Foods: Chemistry Consumption and Health Effects*, New York, Alan R. Liss, 1984, pp. 149–78.

19 M. M. Hetherington and J. I. MacDiarmid, 'Chocolate addiction: a preliminary study of its description and its relationship to problem eating', *Appetite*, 21, 1993, 233–46.

20 D. Benton and K. Greenfield, The development of an Attitudes to Chocolate questionnaire, submitted for publication.

21 P. Rozin, E. Leveine and C. Stoess, 'Chocolate craving and liking', *Appetite*, 17, 1991, 199–212.

22 A. Weil, *Natural Health, Natural Medicine*, Boston, Mass., Houghton Mifflin, 1990.

23 F. Finnigan and R. Hammersley, 'Effects of alcohol on performance', in A. P. Smith and D. M. Jones (eds.), *Handbook of Human Performance*, vol. 2, London, Academic Press, 1992, pp. 73–126.

24 N. Brewer and B. Sandow, 'Alcohol effects on driver performance under conditions of divided attention', *Ergonomics*, 23, 1980, 185–90.

25 R. Radlow and P. M. Hurst, 'Temporal relations between blood alcohol concentration and alcohol effect: an experiment with human subjects', *Psychopharmacology*, 85, 1985, 260–66.

26 K. Millar, R. H. Hammersley and F. Finnigan, 'Reduction of alcohol-induced impairment by prior ingestion of food', *British Journal of Psychology*, 83, 1992, 261–78.

27 Finnigan and Hammersley in Smith and Jones, *Handbook of Human Performance*.

28 J. A. Yesavage and V. O. Leirer, 'Hangover effects on aircraft pilots 14 hours after alcohol ingestion: a preliminary report', *American Journal of Psychiatry*, 143, 1986, 1546–50.

29 *GRAS list survey, Phase III: Estimating distribution of daily intakes of caffeine*, Washington, DC, National Technical Information Service of the National Academy of Sciences, 1978.

30 R. M. Gilbert, 'Caffeine consumption', in G. A. Spiller (ed.), *The*

*Methylxanthine Beverages and Foods: Chemistry Consumption and Health Effects*, New York, Alan R. Liss, 1984, pp. 185–213.

31 H. R. Lieberman, R. J. Wurtman, G. G. Embe, C. Roberts and I. L. G. Coviella, 'The effects of low doses of caffeine on human performance and mood', *Psychopharmacology*, 92, 1987, 308–12.

32 K. Gilliland and D. Andress, 'Ad lib caffeine consumption, symptoms of caffeinism and academic performance', *American Journal of Psychiatry*, 138, 1981, 512–14.

33 I. Karacan, J. I. Thornby, A. M. Anch, G. Booth and R. L. Williams, 'Dose-related sleep disturbances induced by coffee and caffeine', *Journal of Clinical Pharmacology and Therapeutics*, 20, 1976, 682–9.

34 D. L. Costill, G. P. Dalsky and W. J. Fink, 'Effects of caffeine ingestion on metabolism and exercise performance', *Medical Science in Sport*, 10, 1978, 155–8.

35 K. Silverman, S. M. Evans, E. C. Strain and R. R. Griffiths, 'Withdrawal syndrome after the double-blind cessation of caffeine consumption', *The New England Journal of Medicine*, 327, 1992, 1109–14.

36 J. R. Hughes, G. Amori and D. K. Hatsukami, 'A survey of physicians' advice about caffeine', *Journal of Substance Abuse*, 1, 1988, 67–70.

37 R. N. Elkins, J. L. Rapoport, T. B. Zahn, M. S. Buchsbaum, H. Weingartner, I. J. Kopin, D. Langer and C. Johnson, 'Acute effects of caffeine in normal prepubertal boys', *American Journal of Psychiatry*, 138, 1981, 178–83.

38 T. R. Gunn, K. Metrako, P. Riley, D. Willis and J. V. Aranda, 'Sequelae of caffeine treatment in preterm infants with apnea', *Journal of Pediatrics*, 94, 1979, 106–9.

## 13. What Should You Do about Your Diet?

1 R. W. Anderson and A. Lev-Ran, 'Hypoglycemia: the standard and the fiction', *Psychosomatics*, 26, 1985, 38–47.

2 Royal College of Physicians, 'Food intolerance and food aversion', *Journal of the Royal College of Physicians*, 18, 1984, 3–41.

3 P. White, 'Megavitamin this and megavitamin that', *Journal of the American Medical Association*, 233, 1975, 538–9.

4 T. H. Jukes, 'Megavitamin therapy', *Journal of the American Medical Association*, 233, 1975, 550–51.

5 R. J. Williams, *Biochemical Individuality*, New York, John Wiley, 1956.

6 R. Cook and D. Benton, 'Chromium supplementation improves chronic headaches: a case study', *Journal of Nutritional Medicine*, 3, 1992, 61–4.

7 Department of Health and Human Services, *The Surgeon General's report on nutrition and health*, Washington, DC, US Government Printing Office, 1988; National Advisory Committee on Nutrition Education, *Proposal for Nutritional Guidelines for Health Education in Britain*, London, Health Education Council, 1983.

# Index

# READ MORE IN PENGUIN

In every corner of the world, on every subject under the sun, Penguin represents quality and variety – the very best in publishing today.

For complete information about books available from Penguin – including Puffins, Penguin Classics and Arkana – and how to order them, write to us at the appropriate address below. Please note that for copyright reasons the selection of books varies from country to country.

**In the United Kingdom**: Please write to *Dept. EP, Penguin Books Ltd, Bath Road, Harmondsworth, West Drayton, Middlesex UB7 ODA*

**In the United States**: Please write to *Consumer Sales, Penguin USA, P.O. Box 999, Dept. 17109, Bergenfield, New Jersey 07621-0120.* VISA and MasterCard holders call 1-800-253-6476 to order Penguin titles

**In Canada**: Please write to *Penguin Books Canada Ltd, 10 Alcorn Avenue, Suite 300, Toronto, Ontario M4V 3B2*

**In Australia**: Please write to *Penguin Books Australia Ltd, P.O. Box 257, Ringwood, Victoria 3134*

**In New Zealand**: Please write to *Penguin Books (NZ) Ltd, Private Bag 102902, North Shore Mail Centre, Auckland 10*

**In India**: Please write to *Penguin Books India Pvt Ltd, 706 Eros Apartments, 56 Nehru Place, New Delhi 110 019*

**In the Netherlands**: Please write to *Penguin Books Netherlands bv, Postbus 3507, NL-1001 AH Amsterdam*

**In Germany**: Please write to *Penguin Books Deutschland GmbH, Metzlerstrasse 26, 60594 Frankfurt am Main*

**In Spain**: Please write to *Penguin Books S. A., Bravo Murillo 19, 1° B, 28015 Madrid*

**In Italy**: Please write to *Penguin Italia s.r.l., Via Felice Casati 20, I-20124 Milano*

**In France**: Please write to *Penguin France S. A., 17 rue Lejeune, F-31000 Toulouse*

**In Japan**: Please write to *Penguin Books Japan, Ishikiribashi Building, 2-5-4, Suido, Bunkyo-ku, Tokyo 112*

**In Greece**: Please write to *Penguin Hellas Ltd, Dimocritou 3, GR-106 71 Athens*

**In South Africa**: Please write to *Longman Penguin Southern Africa (Pty) Ltd, Private Bag X08, Bertsham 2013*

# READ MORE IN PENGUIN

## A SELECTION OF HEALTH BOOKS

**The Kind Food Guide**   Audrey Eyton

Audrey Eyton's all-time bestselling *The F-Plan Diet* turned the nation on to fibre-rich food. Now, as the tide turns against factory farming, she provides the guide destined to bring in a new era of eating.

**Baby and Child**   Penelope Leach

This comprehensive, authoritative and practical handbook is an essential guide, with sections on every stage of the first five years of life.

**Woman's Experience of Sex**   Sheila Kitzinger

Fully illustrated with photographs and line drawings, this book explores the riches of women's sexuality at every stage of life. 'A book which any mother could confidently pass on to her daughter – and her partner too' – *Sunday Times*

**The Effective Way to Stop Drinking**   Beauchamp Colclough

Beauchamp Colclough is an international authority on drink dependency, a reformed alcoholic, and living proof that today's decision is tomorrow's freedom. Follow the expert advice contained here, and it will help you give up drinking – for good.

**Living with Alzheimer's Disease and Similar Conditions**
Dr Gordon Wilcock

This complete and compassionate self-help guide is designed for families and carers (professional or otherwise) faced with the 'living bereavement' of dementia.

**Living with Stress**
Cary L. Cooper, Rachel D. Cooper and Lynn H. Eaker

Stress leads to more stress, and the authors of this helpful book show why low levels of stress are desirable and how best we can achieve them in today's world. Looking at those most vulnerable, they demonstrate ways of breaking the vicious circle that can ruin lives.

# READ MORE IN PENGUIN

## A SELECTION OF HEALTH BOOKS

**Living with Asthma and Hay Fever** John Donaldson

For the first time, there are now medicines that can prevent asthma attacks from taking place. Based on up-to-date research, this book shows how the majority of sufferers can beat asthma and hay fever to lead full and active lives.

**Anorexia Nervosa** R. L. Palmer

Lucid and sympathetic guidance for those who suffer from this disturbing illness and their families and professional helpers, given with a clarity and compassion that will make anorexia more understandable and consequently less frightening for everyone involved.

**Medicines: A Guide for Everybody** Peter Parish

The use of any medicine is always a balance of benefits and risks – this book will help the reader understand how to extend the benefits and reduce the risks. Completely revised, it is written in ordinary, accessible language for the layperson, and is also indispensable to anyone involved in health care.

**Other People's Children** Sheila Kitzinger

Though step-families are common, adults and children in this situation often feel isolated because they fail to conform to society's idealized picture of a normal family. This sensitive, incisive book is essential reading for anyone involved with or in a step family.

**Miscarriage** Ann Oakley, Ann McPherson and Helen Roberts

One million women worldwide become pregnant every day. At least half of these pregnancies end in miscarriage or stillbirth. But each miscarriage is the loss of a potential baby, and that loss can be painful to adjust to. Here is sympathetic support and up-to-date information on one of the commonest areas of women's reproductive experience.

# READ MORE IN PENGUIN

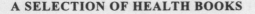

## A SELECTION OF HEALTH BOOKS

**When a Woman's Body Says No to Sex**  Linda Valins

Vaginismus – an involuntary spasm of the vaginal muscles that prevents penetration – has been discussed so little that many women who suffer from it don't recognize their condition by its name. Linda Valins's practical and compassionate guide will liberate these women from their fears and sense of isolation and help them find the right form of therapy.

**Mixed Messages**  Brigid McConville

Images of breasts – young and naked, sexual and chic – are everywhere. Yet for many women, the form, functions and health of our own breasts remain shrouded in mystery, ignorance – even fear. The consequences of our culture's breast taboos are tragic: Britain's breast-cancer death rate is the highest in the world. Every woman should read *Mixed Messages* – the first book to consider the well-being of our breasts in the wider contexts of our lives.

**Defeating Depression**  Tony Lake

Counselling, medication, and the support of friends can all provide invaluable help in relieving depression. But if we are to combat it once and for all, we must face up to perhaps painful truths about our past and take the first steps forward that can eventually transform our lives. This lucid and sensitive book shows us how.

**Freedom and Choice in Childbirth**  Sheila Kitzinger

Undogmatic, honest and compassionate, Sheila Kitzinger's book raises searching questions about the kind of care offered to the pregnant woman – and will help her make decisions and communicate effectively about the kind of birth experience she desires.

**The Complete New Herbal**  Richard Mabey

The new bible for herb users – authoritative, up-to-date, absorbing to read and hugely informative, with practical, clear sections on cultivation and the uses of herbs in daily life, nutrition and healing.

# READ MORE IN PENGUIN

## A SELECTION OF HEALTH BOOKS

**Twins, Triplets and More**  Elizabeth Bryan

This enlightening study of the multiple birth phenomenon covers all aspects of the subject from conception and birth to old age and death. It also offers much comfort and support as well as carefully researched information gained from meeting several thousands of children and their families.

**Meditation for Everybody**  Louis Proto

Meditation means liberation from stress, anxiety and depression. This lucid and readable book by the author of *Self-Healing* describes a variety of meditative practices. From simple breathing exercises to more advanced techniques, there is something here to suit everybody's needs.

**Endometriosis**  Suzie Hayman

Endometriosis is currently surrounded by many damaging myths. Suzie Hayman's pioneering book will set the record straight and provide both sufferers and their doctors with the information necessary for an improved understanding of this frequently puzzling condition.

**The New Our Bodies, Ourselves**
The Boston Women's Health Book Collective

To be used by all generations, *The New Our Bodies, Ourselves* courageously discusses many difficult issues, and is tailored to the needs of women in the 1990s. It provides the most complete advice and information available on women's health care. This British edition is by Angela Phillips and Jill Rakusen.

**Not On Your Own**  Sally Burningham
The MIND Guide to Mental Health

Cutting through the jargon and confusion surrounding the subject of mental health to provide clear explanations and useful information, *Not On Your Own* will enable those with problems – as well as their friends and relatives – to make the best use of available help or find their own ways to cope.

# READ MORE IN PENGUIN

## A SELECTION OF FOOD AND COOKERY BOOKS

**The Fratelli Camisa Cookery Book** Elizabeth Camisa

From antipasti to zabaglione, from the origins of gorgonzola to the storage of salami, an indispensable guide to real Italian home cooking from Elizabeth Camisa of the famous Fratelli Camisa delicatessen in Soho's Berwick Street.

**A Table in Provence** Leslie Forbes

In her latest culinary adventure the bestselling author of *A Table in Tuscany* captures the essence of French Provençal cooking. 'Gives a wonderful flavour of Provence through the recipes and the author's drawings' – *Country Living*

**Far Flung Floyd** Keith Floyd

Keith Floyd's latest culinary odyssey takes him to the far flung East and the exotic flavours of Malaysia, Hong Kong, Vietnam and Thailand. And as ever, the irrepressible Floyd spices his recipes with witty stories, wry observation and a generous pinch of gastronomic wisdom.

**Chinese Food** Kenneth Lo

'From a Chinese breakfast (*congee* rice, pickled eggs, meat wool, jellied and pickled meats, roasted peanuts and "oil stick" doughnuts) to a feast poetically called Autumn on the Lower Yangtze, Mr Lo takes us brilliantly through a cuisine which it is not frivolous to call a civilization' – *Sunday Times*

**The Dinner Party Book** Patricia Lousada

*The Dinner Party Book* hands you the magic key to entertaining without days of panic or last minute butterflies. The magic lies in cooking each course ahead, so that you can enjoy yourself along with your guests.

**Easy Cooking in Retirement** Louise Davies

The mouth-watering recipes in this book are delightfully easy to prepare and involve the least possible fuss to cook and serve.

# READ MORE IN PENGUIN

## A SELECTION OF FOOD AND COOKERY BOOKS

**Traditional Jamaican Cookery**  Norma Benghiat

Reflecting Arawak, Spanish, African, Jewish, English, French, East Indian and Chinese influences, the exciting recipes in this definitive book range from the lavish eating of the old plantocracy to imaginative and ingenious slave and peasant dishes.

**Cooking in a Bedsitter**  Katharine Whitehorn
Completely revised edition

Practical, light-hearted and full of bright ideas, *Cooking in a Bedsitter* will lure you away from the frying pan and tin-opener towards a healthier, more varied range of delicious dishes.

**Simple Vegetarian Meals**  Rosamond Richardson

Vegetarian food offers an exciting range of flavours and textures. It can be light and summery or rich and warming, homely or exotic. In this inspired book Rosamond Richardson explores all these aspects of vegetarian cooking, emphasizing the simplest, freshest dishes that are imaginative, economical and easy to prepare for one or two people.

**Jane Grigson's Fish Book**  Jane Grigson

A new edition of Jane Grigson's imaginative and comprehensive guide to the delights of cooking and eating fish. 'A splendid book ... Most Britishers are rather shy of fish and how to cook it ... This book will change all that' – *Evening Standard*

**Flavours of Greece**  Rosemary Barron

From the sharp olives, the salty feta and the delicate seafood of the first courses to the fragrant honey pastries and luscious figs of the desserts, Greek food offers a feast of variety that changes with the seasons. With wit and enthusiasm Rosemary Barron shows us how to recreate them in our own kitchen, for family meals or when entertaining.

# READ MORE IN PENGUIN

## A SELECTION OF FOOD AND COOKERY BOOKS

**Real Fast Puddings**  Nigel Slater

'Nigel Slater has produced another winner in *Real Fast Puddings* ...
Slater has great flair for flavour combinations and he talks much sense. The
book is snappy and fun' – *Financial Times*. 'Delectable ... Slater is an
unashamed spoon-licker' – *Daily Telegraph*

**Floyd on Spain**  Keith Floyd

'The recipes in *Floyd on Spain* are *wonderful*. The smells of herbs and
onions, tomato sauce and grilled fish rise from the page and you want to
get out, buy a hunk of hake and cook it with potatoes and garlic' – Prue
Leith in the *Sunday Express*

**Simple French Food**  Richard Olney

'There is no other book about food that is anything like it ... essential and
exciting reading for cooks, of course, but it is also a book for eaters ... its
pages brim over with invention' – *Observer*

**English Bread and Yeast Cookery**  Elizabeth David

'Here is a real book, written with authority and enthusiasm – a collection
of history, investigation, comment, recipes' – Jane Grigson

**The Chocolate Book**  Helge Rubinstein

'Fact-filled celebration of the cocoa bean with toothsome recipes from
turkey in chilli and chocolate sauce to brownies and chocolate grog' – *Mail
on Sunday*. 'Crammed with mouth-watering puddings, drinks, cakes and
confectionery' – *Guardian*

**The Cookery of England**  Elisabeth Ayrton

Her fascinating and beautifully compiled history and recipe book of
English cooking from the fifteenth century to the present day is 'a lovely
book, which could restore pride in our English kitchens' – *The Times
Literary Supplement*

# READ MORE IN PENGUIN

## FROM THE COOKERY LIBRARY

**The Legendary Cuisine of Persia**   Margaret Shaida
Winner of the 1993 Glenfiddich Food Book of the Year Award

Persian cuisine is one of the oldest in the world and justly famous for its subtlety and fragrance. Central to the meal are the numerous dishes of rice sprinkled with saffron, some containing almonds, pistachios and raisins, others with vegetables and spices or even occasionally meat, creating a delicious selection of sweet and savoury tastes. 'Exquisite ... both a joy and a precious contribution to the world of gastronomy' – Claudia Roden

**French Provincial Cooking**   Elizabeth David

'It is difficult to think of any home that can do without Elizabeth David's *French Provincial Cooking* ... One could cook for a lifetime on the book alone' – *Observer*. 'Elizabeth David must have done more than anyone for British home cooking in the past twenty-five years'– *Sunday Times*

**A New Book of Middle Eastern Food**   Claudia Roden

'This is one of those rare cookery books that is a work of cultural anthropology and Mrs Roden's standards of scholarship are so high as to ensure that it has permanent value' – *Observer*

**Charcuterie and French Pork Cookery**   Jane Grigson

'Fully comprehensive ... a detailed and enlightening insight into the preparation and cooking of pork. Altogether a unique book' – *Wine and Food*. 'The research is detailed, the recounting lively, the information fascinating' – *The Times*

**The French Family Feast**   Mireille Johnston

Recreate the mouth-watering stews, delicious aromas and warm ambience of a convivial get-together in a traditional French home. 'Mireille Johnston has that rare combination of qualities, exceptional enthusiasm, remarkable taste, a sound knowledge of and the ability to translate kitchen techniques ... a marvellous compendium of fine, easy to understand recipes' – Craig Claiborne

# READ MORE IN PENGUIN

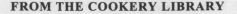

## FROM THE COOKERY LIBRARY

### A Celebration of Soup  Lindsey Bareham

'A rich potage of soups ancient and modern ... looks set to become required bedside reading' – *Independent on Sunday*. 'If you want more soup ideas, *A Celebration of Soup* is a good investment. This is a book about real food, not fashion food; the chapter on stock is masterly' – Frances Bissell in *The Times*

### The Foods and Wines of Spain  Penelope Casas

'I have not come across a book before that captures so well the unlikely medieval mix of Eastern and Northern, earthy and fine, rare and deeply familiar ingredients that make up the Spanish kitchen' – *Harpers and Queen*. 'The definitive book on Spanish cooking ... a jewel in the crown of culinary literature' – Craig Claiborne

### An Omelette and a Glass of Wine  Elizabeth David

'She has the intelligence, subtlety, sensuality, courage and creative force of the true artist' – *Wine and Food*. 'Her pieces are so entertaining, so original, often witty, critical yet lavish with their praise, that they succeed in enthusing even the most jaded palate' – *Vogue*

### English Food  Jane Grigson

'Jane Grigson is perhaps the most serious and discriminating of her generation of cookery writers, and *English Food* is an anthology all who follow her recipes will want to buy for themselves as well as for friends who may wish to know about real English food ... enticing from page to page' – *Spectator*

### Caribbean Cooking  Elisabeth Lambert Ortiz

Caribbean cooking is a delightfully eclectic blend of textures and tastes, influenced by ingredients and cooking techniques from Europe Asia and Africa. Here are tried and tested recipes gathered from Trinidad to the Virgin Islands – carefully ensuring that the more exotic ingredients are easily available.